Emergency Medical Procedures

Designed and edited by

Patient Care Publications, Inc.
Special Publications Group

The procedures in this book have been developed in consultation with:

David G. Eastman, MD
Emergency Physician, Emergency Out-Patient
Department, Frisbie Memorial Hospital,
Rochester, New Hampshire

G. Gordon Snyder, III, MD, FACS
Associate Professor of Surgery and Lecturer,
Emergency Medical Technician (EMT) Program,
University of Connecticut School of Medicine,
Farmington

Kaye E. Wilkins, MD
Clinical Professor of Orthopedics and Pediatrics,
University of Texas Health Science Center,
San Antonio

Additional review and suggestions were
provided by:

**Ad Hoc Committee on Emergency Care
Procedures,** Emergency Department
Nurses Association

Judith West Pronovost, MN, RN
Department of Nursing in Biological
Dysfunction, University of California
School of Nursing, San Francisco

John C. Bechtler, AEMT-P
Coordinator and Senior Instructor
of Emergency Medical Technicians
State of New York Department of Health

Michael G. Dempsey, D.O.
Specialist in Physical Medicine and Rehabilitation
St. Vincent's Hospital and Medical Center of
New York

EMERGENCY MEDICAL PROCEDURES

for the Home, Auto & Workplace

Revised Edition

THE DELTAKRON INSTITUTE

PRENTICE
HALL
PRESS

New York   London   Toronto   Sydney   Tokyo   Singapore

Prentice Hall Press
15 Columbus Circle
New York, New York 10023

Published in 1987 by Prentice Hall Press
A Division of Simon & Schuster, Inc.

This is a revised edition of a book originally
published in 1980 by Prentice-Hall, Inc.

PRENTICE HALL PRESS and colophon are registered
trademarks of Simon & Schuster, Inc.

Library of Congress Catalog Card Number: 86-043098

ISBN: 0-13-274408-2

Manufactured in the United States of America

10 9 8

The information in this book is not intended to replace
instructions by trained professionals. Consult your
local emergency-care personnel or physician if at
all possible before following the author's proposed
courses of emergency treatment. Any application of
the treatments set forth in this book is at the reader's
discretion and sole risk.

Acknowledgments

The Emergency Medical Procedures series has been developed with the assistance of experts in the fields of first aid, nursing, and medicine. We'd like to thank everyone who has consulted on the various segments of this series, including the consultants listed on page i and:

Lynda R. Applegate, MN, FNP; Gordon A. Benner, MD; Shirley F. Boone, RN, MPH; Timothy Burke, EMT; Richard E. Church, MD; Ruth F. Craven, RN, MN; Lance Feild, MA; George Gomez, EMT, RRT; Deanna Grimes, RN, MPH; Greenwich Health Examiners, Inc.; Alan Kallmann, EMS-I, MS; Patricia D. MacDonald, RN, BSN; Marguerite J. Nick, RN; Cornelia P. Porter, RN, MNEd, PNP; John J. Tobin, MD; John Yost, Fire Chief.

The medical information and procedures in this book represent accepted first aid practices adapted and edited for use in the home or while traveling in a car, truck, van, or recreational vehicle. Consideration has been given to possible delays in obtaining medical assistance. All procedures have been reviewed by the participating consultants as well as other experts in first aid, nursing, and medicine.

Contents

^xIntroduction

These emergency medical procedures have been designed to aid you in managing potentially dangerous or troublesome situations at home, at work, or in your car, truck, van, or recreational vehicle. Whether the problem is an illness, injury, or accident, the contents will quickly refer you to a specific problem, but it is a good idea for anyone who may be called upon to use the procedures to read through the material before an emergency occurs to get a general idea of the contents and procedures.

Remember that safety and first aid begin with prevention and that the keys to prevention are health maintenance, a well-balanced diet, and moderate, frequent exercise. It is suggested that you or an appropriate authority:

—Periodically review safety principles and rules, paying special attention to the *Basic Emergency Principles and Transfer Procedures* on p. 2. Include children and sitters in these reviews.

—Be on alert for potentially hazardous situations.

—Assemble a first aid kit to be kept with this book, making sure every employee, family member, and sitter knows where it is. The list on p. 1 includes suggested materials for use with these charts.

—Make sure that you and at least one other person in your household take cardiopulmonary resuscitation (CPR) and annual refresher courses. Your local Heart Association or Red Cross chapter can provide information on these courses.

The following recommendations will help you to prevent potential emergencies or to handle those that may occur at home, at work, or on the road despite your precautions.

At Home and Work

—Contact your local fire and/or police department for instructions on emergency evacuation procedures. In areas where hurricanes, tornadoes, and earthquakes are threats, ask where to obtain information on handling such emergencies. All procedures should be adapted to your particular situation and learned by all family members and sitters. Posting these procedures in a central location, along with this book, also is wise.

—Before an emergency occurs, write emergency phone numbers on pages 55-55A of this book. Post copies of these numbers by every phone. Teach young children the emergency or ambulance number and the fire or police number and how to dial them.

On the Road

—Practice good driving habits: Don't drive when tired or under the influence of alcohol, marijuana, or drugs; and don't rely on caffeine or other stimulants to keep you awake. Stay alert and drive defensively.

—Keep your vehicle in good working condition.

—Limit driving when road conditions are hazardous.

—Make it a rule, particularly when road conditions are hazardous, to note the last emergency call box, home, or open business.

—Assemble a vehicular emergency kit that includes warning lights or flares, a flashlight, emergency signs, and glass cleaner.

—Consider investing in a CB radio if you do not already own one.

—If you live in or are traveling to an area with potentially dangerous climatic or geographical factors, learn and teach others traveling with you how to deal with problems that may arise. For example, in cold weather when confined to a vehicle because of a flat tire, accident, snow, or other reason, use blankets and body heat for warmth; keep the exhaust pipe clear of snow, dirt, and other matter; and run the engine and heater for only 10 minutes every hour. Running the engine more frequently may result in asphyxiation.

—Before an emergency occurs, read *Arrival at the Scene of an Accident* on p. 3.

When a medical emergency occurs:

Remain calm. Take a deep breath, then read these instructions. With all emergencies, except when there is no pulse (then turn immediately to CPR, pp. 8-10), one or two minutes spent getting the situation under control will improve your effectiveness.

Look up the major problem in the Contents. If a serious emergency occurs that you can not find listed, the best procedure is to obtain emergency or medical assistance.

Provide only emergency care outlined in these charts unless you receive instructions for additional care from a medically trained person via telephone, radio, or other means.

Use common sense with these charts; only you know your particular situation. The primary rule of emergency aid is to cause no further injury. Most important during any medical emergency — Remember your ABCs:

— Make sure the *airway* is unobstructed.
— Make sure the person is *breathing*.
— Be sure the *circulation* of blood is maintained.
  (Heart is kept pumping, bleeding is controlled, etc.)

Getting Help

When you are faced with an emergency situation, you will have to use your own judgment about how to get help. When emergency assistance is necessary, you will have to decide, particularly in a vehicular emergency, whether it is best to summon help or drive the person to an emergency room. When a person is sick or injured while riding in a vehicle, you will have to decide also whether the person can be cared for without stopping or whether care can best be given by pulling off the road or to a nearby home or business. When you need additional assistance, whether at home or on the road, use one or more of the following:

— *Telephone:* A telephone is your best means of getting help. On the road, don't forget such sources of telephones as an emergency call box, a home, or an open business.

— *Radio:* Use any two-way radio, such as a CB. On a CB, emergencies are reported on channel 9. On the road, if you don't have a radio, flag down a taxi, delivery truck, or private motorist with a CB.

In addition to the above, the following distress signals may be used and are particularly geared to emergencies which may occur while driving in sparsely populated areas:

— *Standard Ground-to-Air Signals:* As large as possible, illustrate by digging in dirt or snow or use tree limbs, rocks, clothing, etc. Be sure the symbols contrast the ground color as much as possible.

    ▌ for "Require doctor — serious injuries"
    ▌▌ for "Require medical supplies"

— *Universal Distress Signals:* A series of three sights or sounds, such as shouts, blows on a whistle or horn, high-frequency beeps, gunshots, or flashes of light.

— *SOS Morse Code Distress Signal:* A series of three dots, three dashes, three dots made by blows on a whistle or horn, high-frequency beeps, or flashes of light.

    . . . — — — . . . means SOS or Help!

— *A large flag* at the top of a tree or hung on an antenna — the brighter, the better.

— *A mirror or other shiny object* flashed across the sky several times a day to attract planes.

— *Flares*

¹Basic Medical Supplies

Basic Medical Supplies for Use With the Emergency Medical Procedures

The supplies specified are divided into two lists: one consists of medical supplies, which should be kept separate for emergency care and first aid; the other consists of cooking or basic supplies, which may be used for other purposes as well as for emergencies. The designated provisions include only those supplies required in these charts. Most of these items are available in supermarkets or pharmacies.

The two lists should meet the needs for treating injuries or illnesses most frequently encountered in the home, at work, or on the road. However, if anyone in your household, workplace, or vehicle has a history of allergic reaction to insect stings, or if you live, work, or are traveling in an area densely inhabited by insects, we recommend that you include an insect-bite kit, available by prescription from your physician. It is also advisable to include a snakebite kit in regions populated by poisonous snakes.

Many of the suggested materials are marked with an asterisk (*) to indicate that they are not crucial and/or feasible for a *vehicle* medical supply kit. Unless you will be driving in an area that is very isolated, it is assumed that these supplies would be readily obtainable at a nearby home, store, or other business.

Medical Supplies
activated charcoal tablets (medicinal)
adhesive tape (1 inch)
antacids (Gelusil, Maalox, Mylanta)*
antihistamine/decongestant (Contac, Dristan, Sudafed)
aspirin and acetaminophen (Tylenol, Datril)
cold pack
calamine lotion*
cotton swabs*
elastic bandage (3 inch)
Epsom salts*
fever thermometer*
hydrogen peroxide
insect-bite kit**
lip balm (ChapStick, etc.)*
oil of cloves*
petroleum jelly (Vaseline, etc.)*
razor blade*
rubbing alcohol
scissors
smelling salts (ammonia capsules)*
snakebite kit***
sterile gauze bandage (3 inch)
sterile gauze pads (4 x 4 inches)
syrup of ipecac
thermal blanket
topical antibiotic ointment (Triple-Antibiotic Ointment, Neosporin, Bacitracin, etc.)
tweezers
vaporizer (preferably cold-steam)*

Cooking and Basic Supplies that can be used as Medical Supplies
aluminum foil
baking soda
blankets
bouillon cubes
candle or paraffin*
clean cloth (pieces of sheeting)
cup
drinking water*
fruit juices (with sugar added)*
honey*
meat tenderizer*
milk*
plastic bags
plastic wrap
salt
soap (without deodorant, cold cream)*
soft drinks (sugar-sweetened)*
sugar (loose)*
tea*
towels*
wire cutters*

*Not crucial and/or feasible for a *vehicle* medical supply kit unless in a very isolated area.
**If someone is allergic to stings.
***If in an area inhabited by poisonous snakes.

2 Basic Emergency Principles & Transfer Procedures

1. If necessary:

   — Clear mouth and throat of foreign matter to establish and maintain open airway.

   — Check breathing. If it has stopped, begin artificial respiration. (See p. 4.)

   — Check carotid pulse. If no pulse, begin CPR. (See pp. 8-10.)

   — Control bleeding. (See p. 50.)

2. **Do not** move sick or injured person, particularly with back or neck injury, unless:

   — location is dangerous (i.e., fire, threat of explosion, etc.) or

   — crucial emergency care cannot be given at present location.

3. If person is unconscious from direct blow to head or a fall, assume neck, and possibly back, injury. (See p. 29.)

4. — Check for injuries and immobilize all injured parts, if possible.

   — **Do not** straighten fractured or dislocated limbs unless circulation is impaired (i.e. limb turning blue, etc.).

   — **Do not** remove objects imbedded deeply in person (i.e., knife, pencil) and **do not** remove person who is stuck on an object (i.e. fence post, stick shift). Instead, immobilize person and object to prevent further injury. If moving is necessary, disassemble or shorten object and transport person with imbedded object immobilized.

   — Avoid jarring person unnecessarily while preparing for transfer.

   — Always transport person lying down, not in a sitting position.

5. Obtain assistance whenever possible before moving sick or injured person.

Clear airway.

Check carotid pulse.

If possibility of back and/or neck injury, see p. 29.

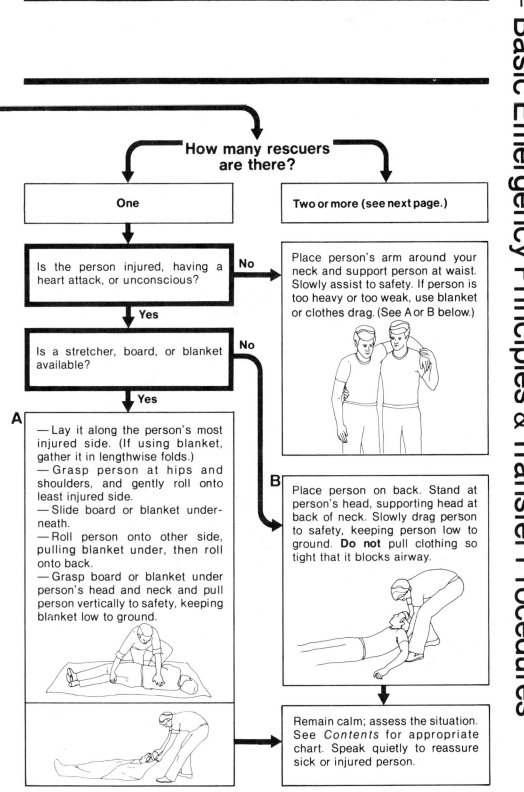

How many rescuers are there?

| One | Two or more (see next page.) |

One:

Is the person injured, having a heart attack, or unconscious? — **No** → Place person's arm around your neck and support person at waist. Slowly assist to safety. If person is too heavy or too weak, use blanket or clothes drag. (See A or B below.)

Yes ↓

Is a stretcher, board, or blanket available? — **No**

Yes ↓

A
— Lay it along the person's most injured side. (If using blanket, gather it in lengthwise folds.)
— Grasp person at hips and shoulders, and gently roll onto least injured side.
— Slide board or blanket underneath.
— Roll person onto other side, pulling blanket under, then roll onto back.
— Grasp board or blanket under person's head and neck and pull person vertically to safety, keeping blanket low to ground.

B
Place person on back. Stand at person's head, supporting head at back of neck. Slowly drag person to safety, keeping person low to ground. **Do not** pull clothing so tight that it blocks airway.

Remain calm; assess the situation. See *Contents* for appropriate chart. Speak quietly to reassure sick or injured person.

Two or more rescuers

Is the person injured, having a heart attack, or unconscious? **Yes** → Is a stretcher, board, or blanket available? **Yes** →

No

No

Place person's arms around each rescuer's neck. Rescuers support person around waist, slightly lifting person, and assist to safety.

— Two rescuers stand on same side of sick or injured person.
— *Rescuer nearest person's feet:* Place one arm under person's knees, and cross other arm over person's hips.
— *Rescuer nearest person's head:* Place arm closest to first rescuer underneath person's hip and grasp other rescuer's hand. Use other arm to support person's neck and back.
— *Third rescuer, if available:* Support person's legs.
— Carry person to safety.

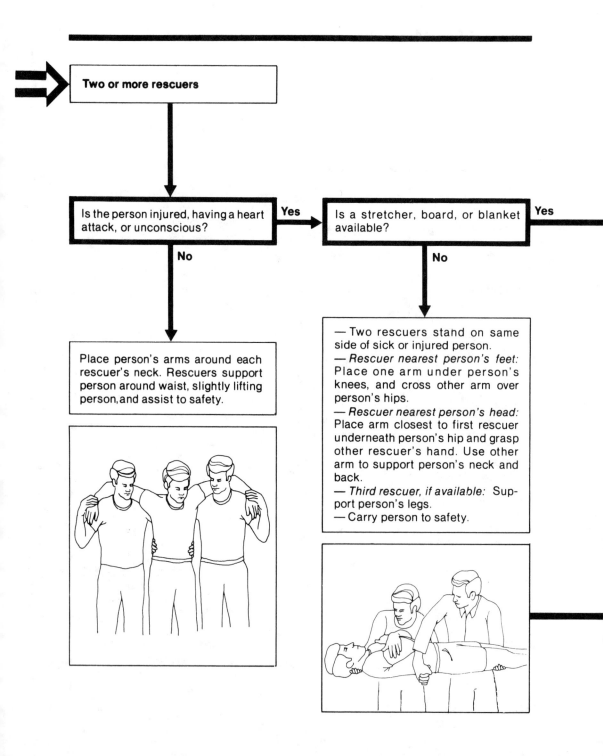

— Lay it along the person's most injured side. (If using blanket, gather it in lengthwise folds.)
— Grasp person at hips and shoulders, and gently roll onto least injured side.
— Slide board underneath, then gently roll person on back.
— Rescuers stand on either side of person, lift slowly and simultaneously, and carry to safety.

Remain calm; assess the situation. See *Contents* for appropriate chart. Speak quietly to reassure sick or injured person.

3 Arrival at the Scene of an Accident
(When assistance has not already arrived)

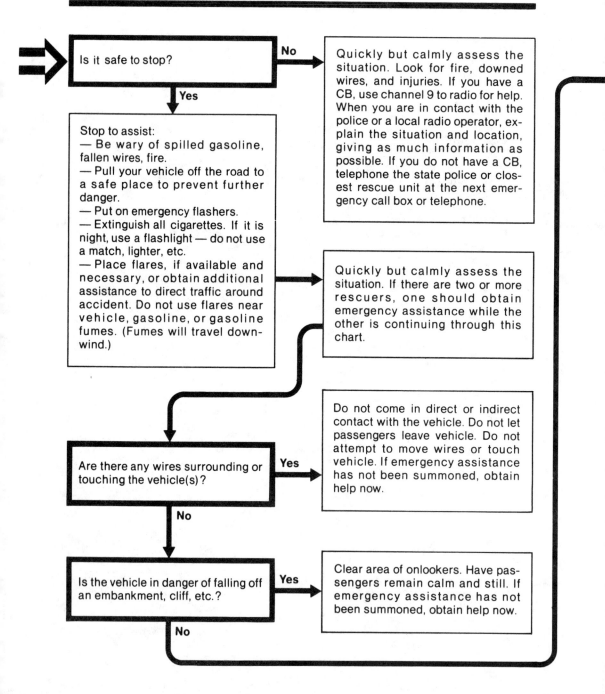

Is it safe to stop? — **No** → Quickly but calmly assess the situation. Look for fire, downed wires, and injuries. If you have a CB, use channel 9 to radio for help. When you are in contact with the police or a local radio operator, explain the situation and location, giving as much information as possible. If you do not have a CB, telephone the state police or closest rescue unit at the next emergency call box or telephone.

Yes ↓

Stop to assist:
— Be wary of spilled gasoline, fallen wires, fire.
— Pull your vehicle off the road to a safe place to prevent further danger.
— Put on emergency flashers.
— Extinguish all cigarettes. If it is night, use a flashlight — do not use a match, lighter, etc.
— Place flares, if available and necessary, or obtain additional assistance to direct traffic around accident. Do not use flares near vehicle, gasoline, or gasoline fumes. (Fumes will travel downwind.)

Quickly but calmly assess the situation. If there are two or more rescuers, one should obtain emergency assistance while the other is continuing through this chart.

Are there any wires surrounding or touching the vehicle(s)? — **Yes** → Do not come in direct or indirect contact with the vehicle. Do not let passengers leave vehicle. Do not attempt to move wires or touch vehicle. If emergency assistance has not been summoned, obtain help now.

No ↓

Is the vehicle in danger of falling off an embankment, cliff, etc.? — **Yes** → Clear area of onlookers. Have passengers remain calm and still. If emergency assistance has not been summoned, obtain help now.

No ↓

Never right an overturned vehicle or do anything else which may cause further injury or danger unless directed to do so below or by trained emergency or medical authorities.

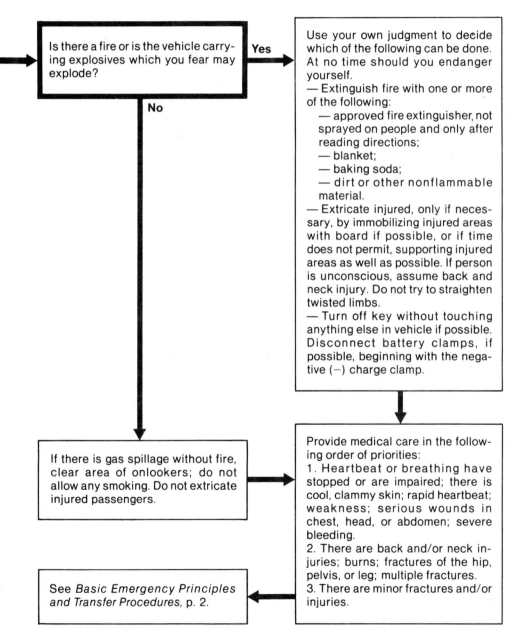

Is there a fire or is the vehicle carrying explosives which you fear may explode?

Yes

No

Use your own judgment to decide which of the following can be done. At no time should you endanger yourself.
— Extinguish fire with one or more of the following:
    — approved fire extinguisher, not sprayed on people and only after reading directions;
    — blanket;
    — baking soda;
    — dirt or other nonflammable material.
— Extricate injured, only if necessary, by immobilizing injured areas with board if possible, or if time does not permit, supporting injured areas as well as possible. If person is unconscious, assume back and neck injury. Do not try to straighten twisted limbs.
— Turn off key without touching anything else in vehicle if possible. Disconnect battery clamps, if possible, beginning with the negative (−) charge clamp.

If there is gas spillage without fire, clear area of onlookers; do not allow any smoking. Do not extricate injured passengers.

Provide medical care in the following order of priorities:
1. Heartbeat or breathing have stopped or are impaired; there is cool, clammy skin; rapid heartbeat; weakness; serious wounds in chest, head, or abdomen; severe bleeding.
2. There are back and/or neck injuries; burns; fractures of the hip, pelvis, or leg; multiple fractures.
3. There are minor fractures and/or injuries.

See *Basic Emergency Principles and Transfer Procedures*, p. 2.

4 Artificial Respiration
(Rescue Breathing)

This chart should only be used if the person is not breathing, but his heart is beating. Check the neck carefully for a carotid pulse; it may be very faint. If the person has no pulse, see *CPR* (p. 8). Artificial respiration should be performed even if a person has been under water for up to 60 minutes. If there is a possibility that the person choked before breathing stopped, see *Choking* (p. 7).

Clear airway. Remove foreign matter with a cloth- or gauze-wrapped finger if necessary. Then turn person on back on a hard surface.

For an adult or older child, use one hand to gently lift person's chin while pushing forehead down with the other hand. **Do not tilt head back if neck is injured.*** *For an infant,* support upper back with hand or folded sheet or towel and gently lift chin forward, **unless neck is injured. Do not over-extend neck.**

For an adult pinch nostrils with fingers of hand resting on forehead. Do not pinch nostrils of an *infant.*

Reposition person's head and repeat 2 breaths. Continue ventilation for *adults* and *older children* at a rate of 1 every 5 seconds — 1 every 3 seconds for infants, checking carotid pulse every 1-2 minutes, until the person breathes regularly without assistance.

Feel the neck for 5-10 seconds for a carotid pulse. If there is none, see *CPR* (p. 8).

Blow 2 full breaths ($1\frac{1}{2}$ seconds per breath). *For an infant,* blow only small puffs of air. Release your mouth between breaths. If the chest does not rise, make sure all foreign matter and secretions have been removed and *for an adult only,* be sure the head is tilted back to maximum extension, unless neck is injured.

Continue to lift *chin,* take a deep breath, and seal your mouth tightly around person's mouth or over nose and mouth in infants.

If gas or smoke is present, move person to safety.

The first thing you must do if the person appears unconscious is to determine unresponsiveness by shaking the person while asking, "Are you okay?" If the person does not respond, shout for help even if you think you are alone. If there are two or more rescuers, one should obtain emergency assistance while the other is following the procedures outlined below.

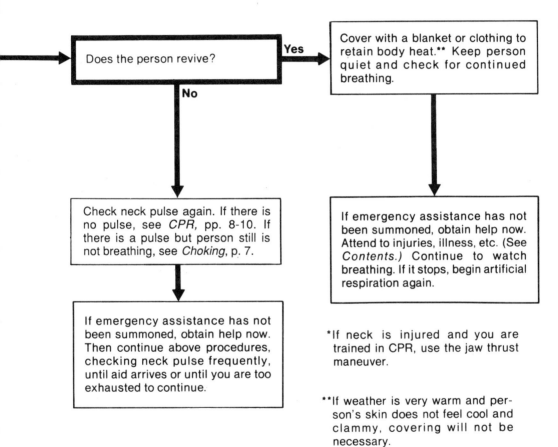

Does the person revive?

Yes — Cover with a blanket or clothing to retain body heat.** Keep person quiet and check for continued breathing.

No

Check neck pulse again. If there is no pulse, see *CPR*, pp. 8-10. If there is a pulse but person still is not breathing, see *Choking*, p. 7.

If emergency assistance has not been summoned, obtain help now. Then continue above procedures, checking neck pulse frequently, until aid arrives or until you are too exhausted to continue.

If emergency assistance has not been summoned, obtain help now. Attend to injuries, illness, etc. (See *Contents*.) Continue to watch breathing. If it stops, begin artificial respiration again.

*If neck is injured and you are trained in CPR, use the jaw thrust maneuver.

**If weather is very warm and person's skin does not feel cool and clammy, covering will not be necessary.

5 Childbirth
(Delivery)

Do not try to slow or speed delivery. Do not let the woman cross her legs or go to the bathroom. Do not place anything into the birth canal. Once you decide there is not enough time to reach the hospital, call for emergency assistance and a physician, or, if impossible, someone who has assisted in childbirth. Follow the procedures outlined below while awaiting assistance.

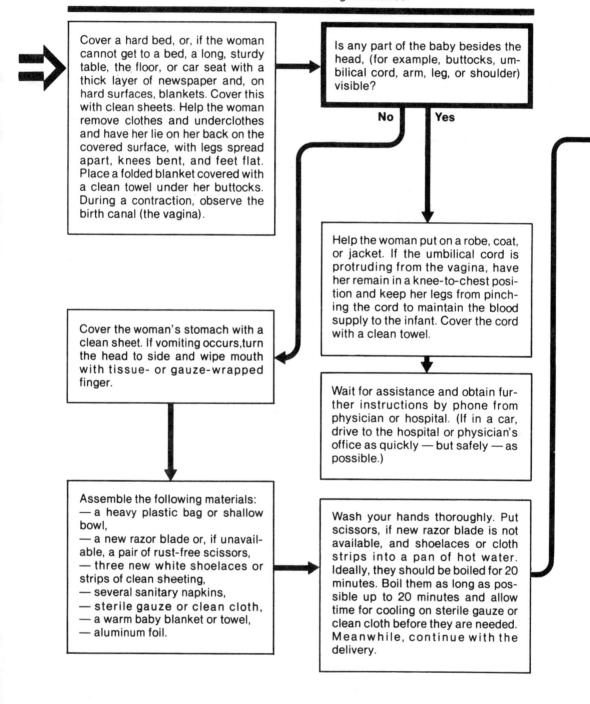

Cover a hard bed, or, if the woman cannot get to a bed, a long, sturdy table, the floor, or car seat with a thick layer of newspaper and, on hard surfaces, blankets. Cover this with clean sheets. Help the woman remove clothes and underclothes and have her lie on her back on the covered surface, with legs spread apart, knees bent, and feet flat. Place a folded blanket covered with a clean towel under her buttocks. During a contraction, observe the birth canal (the vagina).

Is any part of the baby besides the head, (for example, buttocks, umbilical cord, arm, leg, or shoulder) visible?

No   **Yes**

Help the woman put on a robe, coat, or jacket. If the umbilical cord is protruding from the vagina, have her remain in a knee-to-chest position and keep her legs from pinching the cord to maintain the blood supply to the infant. Cover the cord with a clean towel.

Cover the woman's stomach with a clean sheet. If vomiting occurs, turn the head to side and wipe mouth with tissue- or gauze-wrapped finger.

Wait for assistance and obtain further instructions by phone from physician or hospital. (If in a car, drive to the hospital or physician's office as quickly — but safely — as possible.)

Assemble the following materials:
— a heavy plastic bag or shallow bowl,
— a new razor blade or, if unavailable, a pair of rust-free scissors,
— three new white shoelaces or strips of clean sheeting,
— several sanitary napkins,
— sterile gauze or clean cloth,
— a warm baby blanket or towel,
— aluminum foil.

Wash your hands thoroughly. Put scissors, if new razor blade is not available, and shoelaces or cloth strips into a pan of hot water. Ideally, they should be boiled for 20 minutes. Boil them as long as possible up to 20 minutes and allow time for cooling on sterile gauze or clean cloth before they are needed. Meanwhile, continue with the delivery.

Calm the woman by talking while attending to the problem. Explain what you are doing. Try not to show anxiety; act with confidence. Your calm behavior can help to reassure the woman.

If childbirth is imminent while driving, follow these procedures as closely as possible; do not worry if some materials are not available.

As the baby's head emerges, guide and support the baby's head through the birth canal, keeping it free of blood and fluid. Do not pull or twist the head, but exert just enough pressure to keep it from popping out suddenly. If the baby is still inside the bag of waters, tear the bag open to prevent suffocation. The baby's head may be face down and, upon emerging, may turn to the side. If it does not, do not be alarmed.

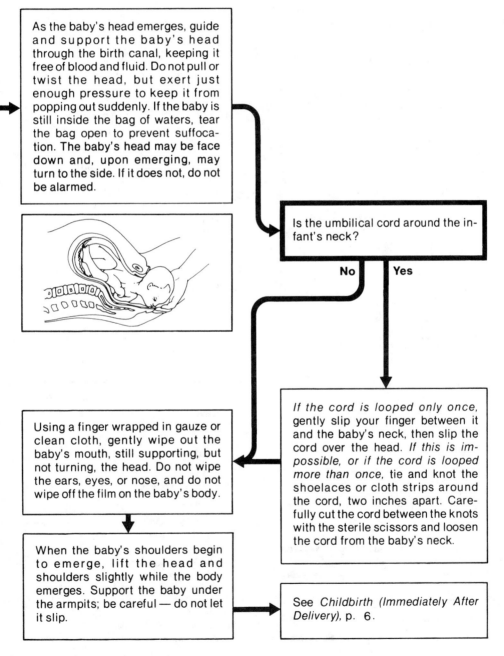

Is the umbilical cord around the infant's neck?

No   **Yes**

Using a finger wrapped in gauze or clean cloth, gently wipe out the baby's mouth, still supporting, but not turning, the head. Do not wipe the ears, eyes, or nose, and do not wipe off the film on the baby's body.

If the cord is looped only once, gently slip your finger between it and the baby's neck, then slip the cord over the head. *If this is impossible, or if the cord is looped more than once,* tie and knot the shoelaces or cloth strips around the cord, two inches apart. Carefully cut the cord between the knots with the sterile scissors and loosen the cord from the baby's neck.

When the baby's shoulders begin to emerge, lift the head and shoulders slightly while the body emerges. Support the baby under the armpits; be careful — do not let it slip.

See *Childbirth (Immediately After Delivery),* p. 6.

6Childbirth
(Immediately After Delivery)

You have just delivered a baby. (See *Childbirth* [Delivery], p. 5.)

Place the baby on its side on a warm blanket or towel. Slap the sole of its foot with a finger several times.

Does the baby begin to breathe? — **No** →

Wipe out mouth and under nose again with gauze or clean cloth. Blow quick, small puffs of air into nose and mouth, at a rate of 1 every 5 seconds. Continue until the baby is breathing well. If breathing does not begin after 2 minutes, check for a pulse above the left nipple. If no pulse, see *CPR (Infants),* p. 10. If there is a pulse, continue giving small puffs of air until breathing begins, checking pulse periodically.

Yes

Cover the baby's arms and legs with the blanket or towel. Place the baby between the mother's legs. If the cord has not been cut, wait until all pulsations have stopped. *If at home,* take the shoelaces or cloth strips and tie one 6 inches from the baby, then tie the other 3 inches beyond the first. Cut the cord between the knots. *If in a car,* do not tie and cut cord.

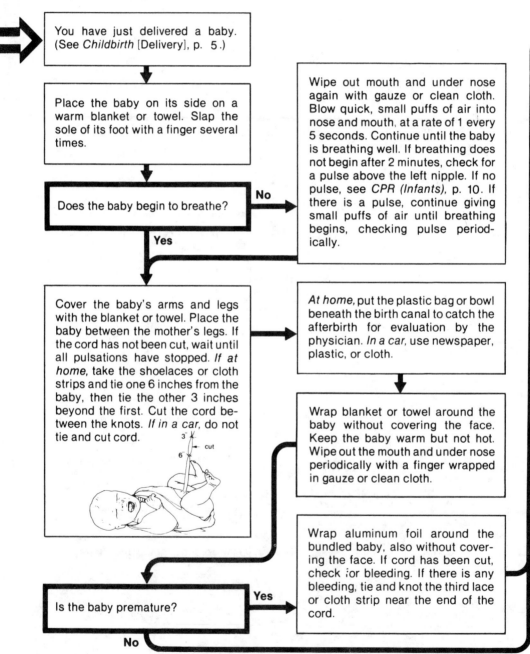

At home, put the plastic bag or bowl beneath the birth canal to catch the afterbirth for evaluation by the physician. *In a car,* use newspaper, plastic, or cloth.

Wrap blanket or towel around the baby without covering the face. Keep the baby warm but not hot. Wipe out the mouth and under nose periodically with a finger wrapped in gauze or clean cloth.

Wrap aluminum foil around the bundled baby, also without covering the face. If cord has been cut, check for bleeding. If there is any bleeding, tie and knot the third lace or cloth strip near the end of the cord.

Is the baby premature? — **Yes** →

No

Calm the woman by talking while attending to the problem. Explain what you are doing. Try not to show anxiety; act with confidence. Your calm behavior can help to reassure the woman.

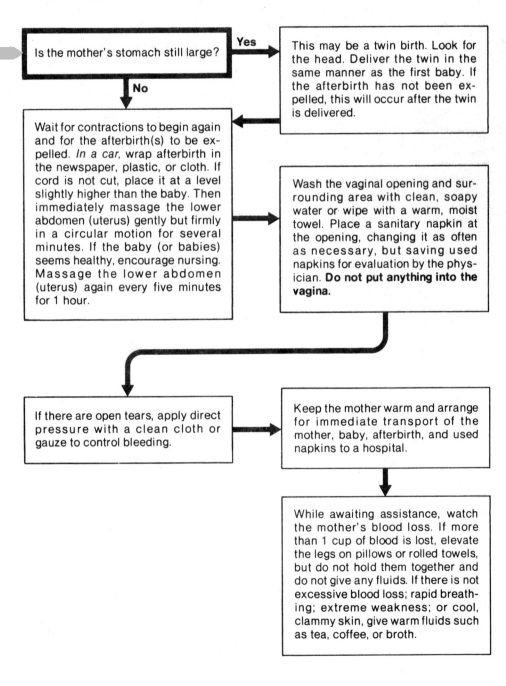

Is the mother's stomach still large?

Yes → This may be a twin birth. Look for the head. Deliver the twin in the same manner as the first baby. If the afterbirth has not been expelled, this will occur after the twin is delivered.

No

Wait for contractions to begin again and for the afterbirth(s) to be expelled. *In a car,* wrap afterbirth in the newspaper, plastic, or cloth. If cord is not cut, place it at a level slightly higher than the baby. Then immediately massage the lower abdomen (uterus) gently but firmly in a circular motion for several minutes. If the baby (or babies) seems healthy, encourage nursing. Massage the lower abdomen (uterus) again every five minutes for 1 hour.

Wash the vaginal opening and surrounding area with clean, soapy water or wipe with a warm, moist towel. Place a sanitary napkin at the opening, changing it as often as necessary, but saving used napkins for evaluation by the physician. **Do not put anything into the vagina.**

If there are open tears, apply direct pressure with a clean cloth or gauze to control bleeding.

Keep the mother warm and arrange for immediate transport of the mother, baby, afterbirth, and used napkins to a hospital.

While awaiting assistance, watch the mother's blood loss. If more than 1 cup of blood is lost, elevate the legs on pillows or rolled towels, but do not hold them together and do not give any fluids. If there is not excessive blood loss; rapid breathing; extreme weakness; or cool, clammy skin, give warm fluids such as tea, coffee, or broth.

7 Choking

Signs & Symptoms: Clutching throat/initial coughing with gasping followed by inability to cough, speak, or breathe while eating/blue or gray skin/loss of consciousness.

Do not use this procedure if person is able to cough or make any noise. **If the person has been injured,** do not move unless necessary.

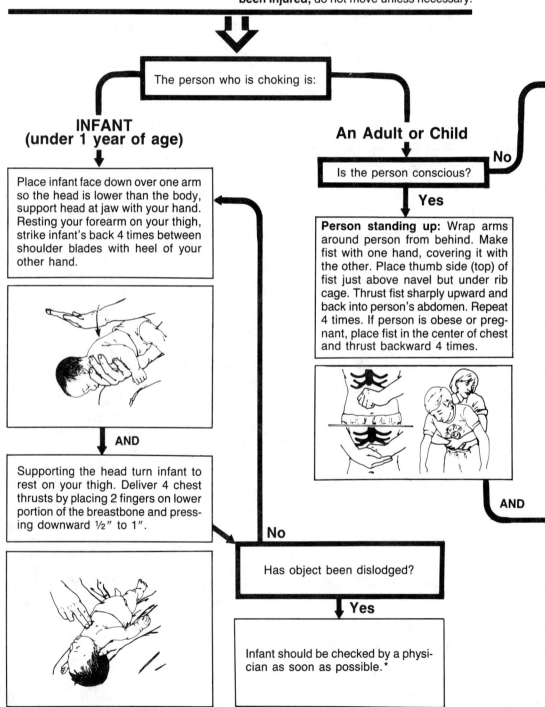

The person who is choking is:

INFANT (under 1 year of age)

Place infant face down over one arm so the head is lower than the body, support head at jaw with your hand. Resting your forearm on your thigh, strike infant's back 4 times between shoulder blades with heel of your other hand.

AND

Supporting the head turn infant to rest on your thigh. Deliver 4 chest thrusts by placing 2 fingers on lower portion of the breastbone and pressing downward ½″ to 1″.

An Adult or Child

Is the person conscious?   **No**

Yes

Person standing up: Wrap arms around person from behind. Make fist with one hand, covering it with the other. Place thumb side (top) of fist just above navel but under rib cage. Thrust fist sharply upward and back into person's abdomen. Repeat 4 times. If person is obese or pregnant, place fist in the center of chest and thrust backward 4 times.

AND

No

Has object been dislodged?

Yes

Infant should be checked by a physician as soon as possible.*

If person was not eating, clutches chest, or indicates there is extreme chest pain, see *Chest Pain,* p. 13.

Shout for help even if you think you are alone. If there are two or more rescuers, one should obtain emergency assistance while the other is following the procedures outlined below.

Person lying down: Straddle the victim. Turn person face up. Cross flat hands and place slightly above navel, but below rib cage. Thrust heel of bottom hand into abdomen with quick upward thrust. Repeat 4 times. If person vomits, immediately wipe out mouth with your fingers.

AND

Kneeling, turn person onto side, facing you with chest against your thigh. Deliver 4 sharp blows to the back with heel of hand over spine between shoulder blades.

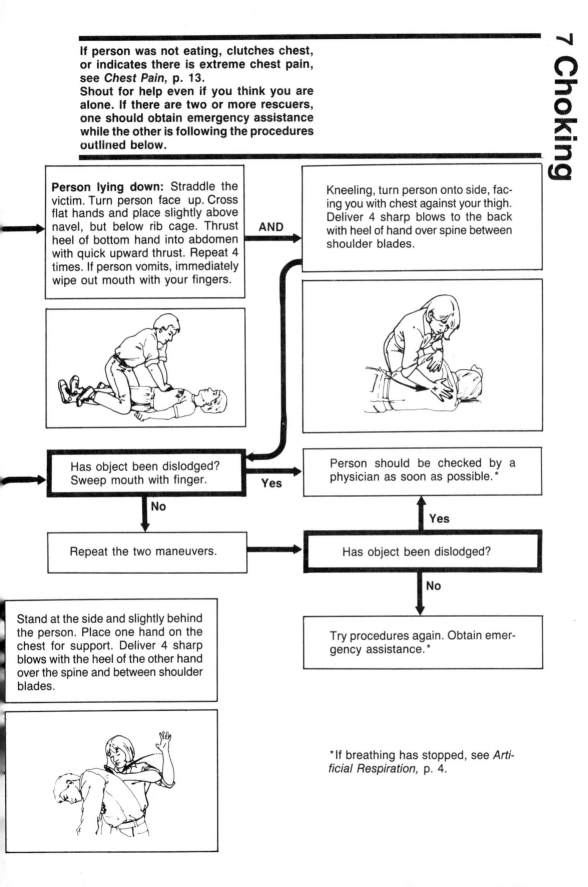

Has object been dislodged? Sweep mouth with finger.

Yes

Person should be checked by a physician as soon as possible. *

No

Repeat the two maneuvers.

Has object been dislodged?

Yes

No

Try procedures again. Obtain emergency assistance. *

Stand at the side and slightly behind the person. Place one hand on the chest for support. Deliver 4 sharp blows with the heel of the other hand over the spine and between shoulder blades.

*If breathing has stopped, see *Artificial Respiration,* p. 4.

8 CPR
(1 Rescuer)

For infants, see *CPR (Infants)*. p. 10.

If 2 or more rescuers, see p. 9. Begin CPR immediately. Do not use CPR on a person whose heart is beating. It may cause serious complications. Check the neck artery carefully; pulse may be weak. If there is a heartbeat but no sign of breathing, see *Artificial Respiration.* (p. 4).

Place person flat on back on floor or ground. Ask "Are you all right?" two or three times. If person is not aroused, lightly shake or slap. Shout for help, even if you think you are alone.

Kneel at side of head. Clear airway. Remove any foreign materials from mouth and gently lift chin while pushing forehead down with other hand. **Do not push head back if neck is injured.***

Pinch nostrils together and rest palm of hand on forehead. Take a deep breath and seal your lips tightly over mouth. Blow 2 deep, full breaths, releasing mouth after each breath.

Feel for pulse for 5-10 seconds. Check the neck artery carefully; pulse may be weak. If there is a pulse, but breathing is weak or absent, continue only ventilation at a rate of 1 every 5 seconds until person revives.

If no pulse, follow ribcage up to center of chest. Place index and middle finger on tip of breastbone.

Place heel of other hand immediately next to and touching the index finger.

For adults, and children over 80 pounds only, place heel of the first hand directly over the wrist of the other hand on the person's lower breastbone. Clasp fingers and bend those of lower hand back. *For children under 80 pounds,* use only heel of one hand.

Lean directly over the person and straighten your arm(s).

adult

small child

Although the necessary fundamentals for performing CPR are set forth on this chart, there is no substitute for a course in CPR given by a certified instructor.

Use straight-down pressure through both arms (one arm for child under 80 pounds) to push breastbone against heart. *For an adult*, depress breastbone 1 1/2'' to 2''; *for a child*, 3/4'' to 1 1/2''.

The compression/relaxation combination is performed at a rate of 80-100 times per minute. Count one-and-two-and-three, etc. Completely release pressure during relaxation phase without lifting your hand(s) from person's chest.

After 15 compressions, breathe twice into the mouth. Repeat the 15-to-2 cycle 4 times.

Are breathing and pulse restored?

No

Check breathing and neck pulse carefully. If no pulse, continue CPR. Check for pulse and breathing every 4-6 cycles until the person is revived, help arrives, or you can no longer continue. If there is a pulse, but breathing is weak or absent, continue only ventilation at a rate of 1 every 5 seconds until person revives. Continue to monitor pulse closely.

Yes

Loosen clothing to relieve pressure. Keep person warm and check for continued breathing and pulse.

If emergency assistance has not been summoned, obtain help now. Attend to injuries, illness, etc. (See *Contents*.)

*If neck is injured and you are trained in CPR, use jaw thrust maneuver.

9 CPR

(2 or More Rescuers)

For infants, see *CPR (Infants)*, p.10.

If only one rescuer, see p. 8. Rescuers read through chart before beginning CPR. If 3 or more rescuers, 2 begin CPR while the other obtains emergency assistance. Rescuers kneel at opposite side of person; one at chest, one at head.

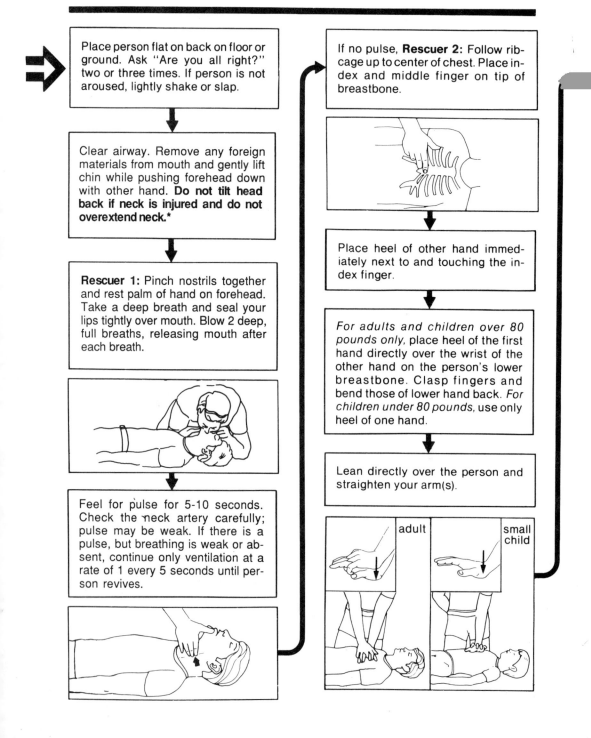

Place person flat on back on floor or ground. Ask "Are you all right?" two or three times. If person is not aroused, lightly shake or slap.

Clear airway. Remove any foreign materials from mouth and gently lift chin while pushing forehead down with other hand. **Do not tilt head back if neck is injured and do not overextend neck.***

Rescuer 1: Pinch nostrils together and rest palm of hand on forehead. Take a deep breath and seal your lips tightly over mouth. Blow 2 deep, full breaths, releasing mouth after each breath.

Feel for pulse for 5-10 seconds. Check the neck artery carefully; pulse may be weak. If there is a pulse, but breathing is weak or absent, continue only ventilation at a rate of 1 every 5 seconds until person revives.

If no pulse, **Rescuer 2:** Follow ribcage up to center of chest. Place index and middle finger on tip of breastbone.

Place heel of other hand immediately next to and touching the index finger.

For adults and children over 80 pounds only, place heel of the first hand directly over the wrist of the other hand on the person's lower breastbone. Clasp fingers and bend those of lower hand back. *For children under 80 pounds,* use only heel of one hand.

Lean directly over the person and straighten your arm(s).

adult

small child

Begin CPR immediately. Do not use CPR on a person whose heart is beating. It may cause serious complications. Check neck artery carefully; pulse may be weak. If there is a heartbeat but no sign of breathing, see *Artificial Respiration* (p. 4.)

Although the necessary fundamentals for performing CPR are set forth on this chart, there is no substitute for a course in CPR given by a certified instructor.

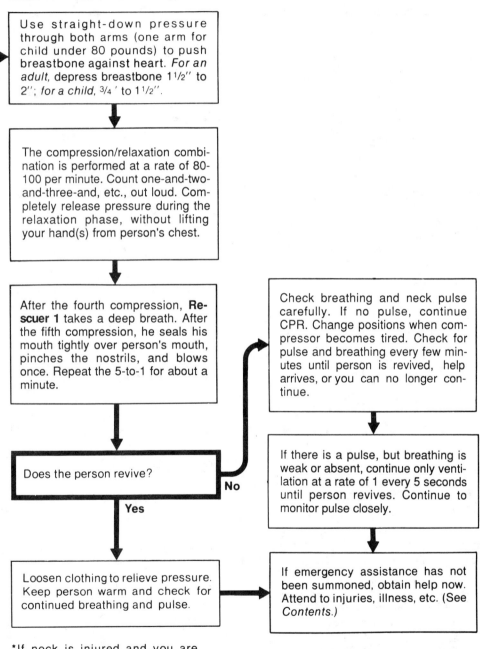

Use straight-down pressure through both arms (one arm for child under 80 pounds) to push breastbone against heart. *For an adult,* depress breastbone 1½" to 2"; *for a child,* ¾' to 1½".

The compression/relaxation combination is performed at a rate of 80-100 per minute. Count one-and-two-and-three-and, etc., out loud. Completely release pressure during the relaxation phase, without lifting your hand(s) from person's chest.

After the fourth compression, **Rescuer 1** takes a deep breath. After the fifth compression, he seals his mouth tightly over person's mouth, pinches the nostrils, and blows once. Repeat the 5-to-1 for about a minute.

Check breathing and neck pulse carefully. If no pulse, continue CPR. Change positions when compressor becomes tired. Check for pulse and breathing every few minutes until person is revived, help arrives, or you can no longer continue.

Does the person revive?

No

Yes

If there is a pulse, but breathing is weak or absent, continue only ventilation at a rate of 1 every 5 seconds until person revives. Continue to monitor pulse closely.

Loosen clothing to relieve pressure. Keep person warm and check for continued breathing and pulse.

If emergency assistance has not been summoned, obtain help now. Attend to injuries, illness, etc. (See *Contents.*)

*If neck is injured and you are trained in CPR, use jaw thrust maneuver.

10 CPR
(Infants)

Begin CPR immediately. If 2 or more rescuers, 1 begin CPR while other gets help. Do not use CPR on an infant whose heart is beating: It may cause serious complications. Check carefully above left nipple for heartbeat; pulse may be weak. If there is a heartbeat but no sign of breathing, see **Artificial Respiration, p. 4.**

Place infant flat on back. Call child's name two or three times; try to arouse by lightly shaking or tapping hard on bottom of bare foot. Shout for help even if you think you are alone.

Clear airway. Remove any foreign material from mouth and gently lift chin slightly, supporting upper back with hand or folded sheet or towel. Do not tilt head back if neck is injured and **do not overextend neck.***

Seal your mouth over infant's mouth and nose and blow 2 puffs of air.

Feel for pulse above left nipple for 5-10 seconds. Check carefully; pulse may be weak. If there is a pulse, but breathing is weak or absent, continue only ventilation at a rate of 1 every 3 seconds until infant revives.

If no pulse, spread one hand over chest so that thumb is at base of throat and little finger is at end of breastbone. Keep index finger and middle finger together and lift others from chest.

With tips of index finger and middle finger press gently on center of breastbone, depressing 1/2" to 3/4"

The compression/relaxation combination is performed at a rate of 80-100 times per minute Count 1-2-3, etc.

Although the necessary fundamentals for performing CPR are set forth on this chart, there is no substitute for a course in CPR given by a certified instructor.

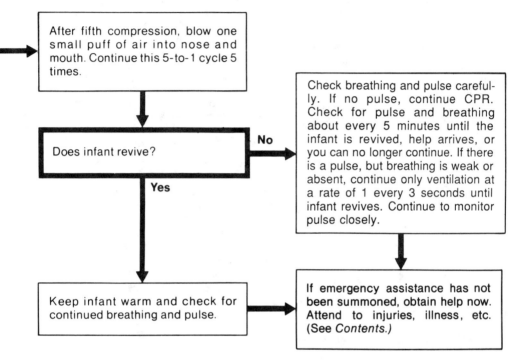

After fifth compression, blow one small puff of air into nose and mouth. Continue this 5-to-1 cycle 5 times.

Does infant revive?

No

Yes

Check breathing and pulse carefully. If no pulse, continue CPR. Check for pulse and breathing about every 5 minutes until the infant is revived, help arrives, or you can no longer continue. If there is a pulse, but breathing is weak or absent, continue only ventilation at a rate of 1 every 3 seconds until infant revives. Continue to monitor pulse closely.

Keep infant warm and check for continued breathing and pulse.

If emergency assistance has not been summoned, obtain help now. Attend to injuries, illness, etc. (See *Contents.*)

*If neck is injured and you are trained in CPR, use the jaw thrust maneuver.

11 Abdominal Pain

Abdominal pain should never be taken lightly. Keep person lying quietly. Do not apply heat to abdomen.

If you suspect *Chemical Poisoning*, see p. 32.

Ask about or check for the following symptoms or conditions. Does the person have . . .

Sharp or burning pain in mid-upper abdominal region, with:
— pain radiating to arm(s), neck, jaw, chest, or to back between shoulder blades?
— difficulty breathing?
— skin, lips, or nails pale or bluish?

Yes →

— Have the person lie back with pillows or rolled blanket behind head and shoulders.
— If this is a heart patient with nitroglycerin or amyl nitrite, give medication as directed on label.
— Loosen clothing. Provide good ventilation. Cover with a light blanket to retain body heat.*
— Obtain emergency assistance.
— While awaiting assistance, watch breathing. If it stops, see *Artificial Respiration*, p. 4.

No ↓

Sharp or burning pain in mid-upper abdominal region with none of the above?

Yes →

Problem may be indigestion, gastritis, or ulcer.
— Give antacids or milk.
— Do not give coffee, tea, alcohol, or aspirin-containing remedies for 24 hours.
If pain persists more than one hour or other symptoms occur, seek medical care.

↓

If pain subsides, have person eat only light foods (soups, broths, etc.) for 24 hours, then gradually return to normal diet. If symptoms recur, seek medical care as soon as possible.

No ↓

Diabetes, with:
— flushed face?
— lethargy, drowsiness?
— hot, dry skin?
— deep, rapid breathing?
— fruity breath odor?
— thirst?

Yes →

See *Diabetic Emergencies*, p. 16 .

No ↓

— Hard and rigid belly?
— Bloody or "coffee grounds" vomit with no recent abdominal injury?
— Bloody or "currant jelly" diarrhea?

Yes →

See *Internal Bleeding*, p. 19 .

No

Calm the person by talking while attending to the problem. Explain what you are doing. Try not to show anxiety; act with confidence. Your calm behavior can help to reassure the sick person.

Open abdominal wound or abdominal injury with:
— swelling and discoloration?
— cold, clammy, pale skin?
— blood in vomit or sputum?
— blood in urine or feces?
— painful mass in groin or scrotum?

Yes → See *Abdominal Injury*, p. 25.

No

Pain and other symptoms within 36 hours of eating mushrooms, plants, shellfish, or questionable foods?

Yes → See *Food Poisoning*, p. 40.

No

Fever or chills?

Yes → See *Fever*, p. 17.

No

Is pain getting worse and/or has it lasted longer than 2 hours?

Yes → Make person comfortable. Seek medical care. If care will be delayed, cover with a blanket to retain body heat.*

No

Problem may be self-limiting. Watch for return of pain or development of other symptoms.

→ If pain does not return and person is feeling better, give light foods (soups, broths, etc.) and water, tea, or soft drinks. Avoid coffee or alcohol and aspirin-containing medications. Continue for 24 hours.

*If weather is very warm and person's skin does not feel cool and clammy, covering will not be necessary.

Asthma Attack

Signs & Symptoms: *wheezing/difficulty breathing/exhaling much more difficult than inhaling/rapid heartbeat/possible hard, tight cough/possible nasal congestion/possible pale, bluish skin, lips, and nails.*

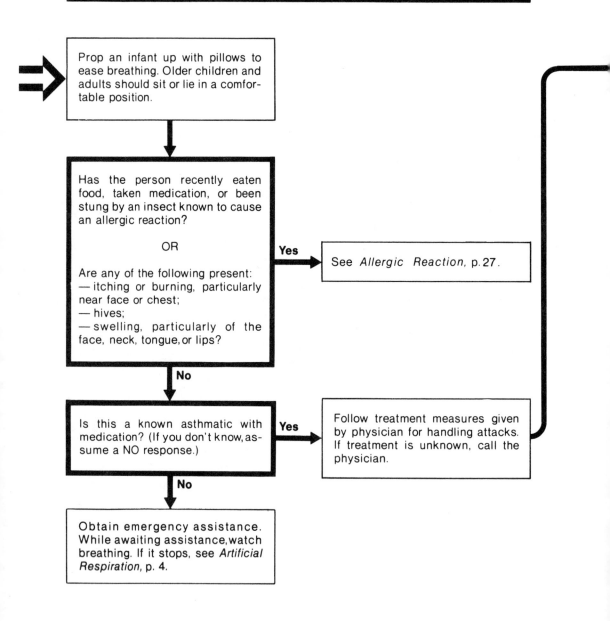

Prop an infant up with pillows to ease breathing. Older children and adults should sit or lie in a comfortable position.

Has the person recently eaten food, taken medication, or been stung by an insect known to cause an allergic reaction?

OR

Are any of the following present:
— itching or burning, particularly near face or chest;
— hives;
— swelling, particularly of the face, neck, tongue, or lips?

Yes → See *Allergic Reaction*, p. 27.

No

Is this a known asthmatic with medication? (If you don't know, assume a NO response.)

Yes → Follow treatment measures given by physician for handling attacks. If treatment is unknown, call the physician.

No

Obtain emergency assistance. While awaiting assistance, watch breathing. If it stops, see *Artificial Respiration*, p. 4.

Calm the person by talking while attending to the problem. Explain what you are doing. Try not to show anxiety; act with confidence. Your calm behavior can help to reassure the sick person.

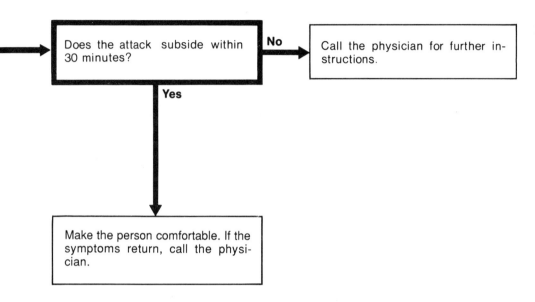

Does the attack subside within 30 minutes?

No

Call the physician for further instructions.

Yes

Make the person comfortable. If the symptoms return, call the physician.

13 Chest Pain

Most chest pain is caused by indigestion or muscular strain. If it is severe, persistent, or worrisome, check symptoms below for more serious ailments.

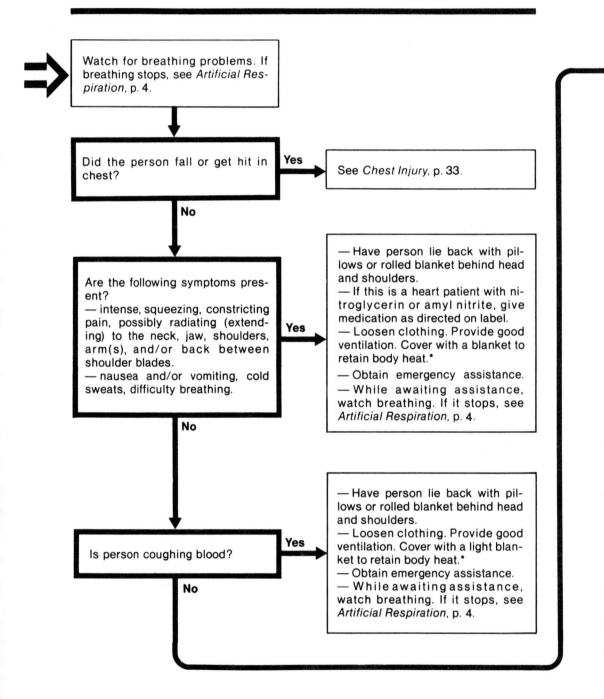

Watch for breathing problems. If breathing stops, see *Artificial Respiration*, p. 4.

Did the person fall or get hit in chest? **Yes** → See *Chest Injury*, p. 33.

No

Are the following symptoms present?
— intense, squeezing, constricting pain, possibly radiating (extending) to the neck, jaw, shoulders, arm(s), and/or back between shoulder blades.
— nausea and/or vomiting, cold sweats, difficulty breathing.

Yes →
— Have person lie back with pillows or rolled blanket behind head and shoulders.
— If this is a heart patient with nitroglycerin or amyl nitrite, give medication as directed on label.
— Loosen clothing. Provide good ventilation. Cover with a blanket to retain body heat.*
— Obtain emergency assistance.
— While awaiting assistance, watch breathing. If it stops, see *Artificial Respiration*, p. 4.

No

Is person coughing blood? **Yes** →
— Have person lie back with pillows or rolled blanket behind head and shoulders.
— Loosen clothing. Provide good ventilation. Cover with a light blanket to retain body heat.*
— Obtain emergency assistance.
— While awaiting assistance, watch breathing. If it stops, see *Artificial Respiration*, p. 4.

No

Calm the person by talking while attending to the problem. Explain what you are doing. Try not to show anxiety; act with confidence. Your calm behavior can help to reassure the sick person.

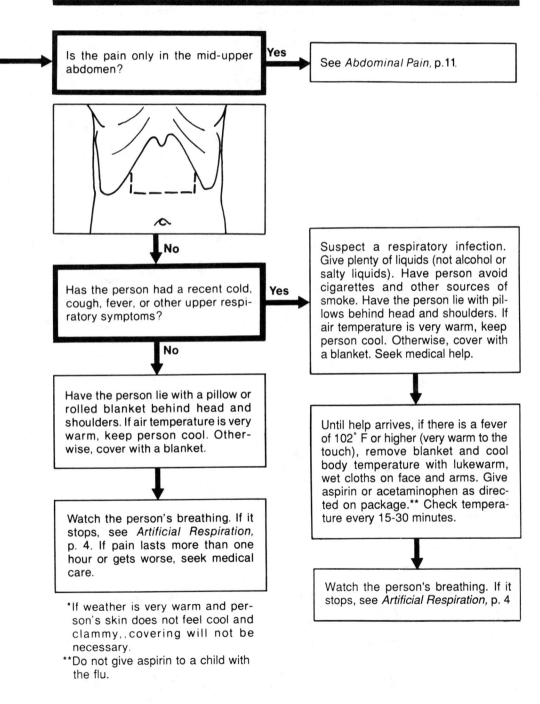

Is the pain only in the mid-upper abdomen?

Yes → See *Abdominal Pain*, p.11.

No

Has the person had a recent cold, cough, fever, or other upper respiratory symptoms?

Yes → Suspect a respiratory infection. Give plenty of liquids (not alcohol or salty liquids). Have person avoid cigarettes and other sources of smoke. Have the person lie with pillows behind head and shoulders. If air temperature is very warm, keep person cool. Otherwise, cover with a blanket. Seek medical help.

No

Have the person lie with a pillow or rolled blanket behind head and shoulders. If air temperature is very warm, keep person cool. Otherwise, cover with a blanket.

Watch the person's breathing. If it stops, see *Artificial Respiration*, p. 4. If pain lasts more than one hour or gets worse, seek medical care.

Until help arrives, if there is a fever of 102° F or higher (very warm to the touch), remove blanket and cool body temperature with lukewarm, wet cloths on face and arms. Give aspirin or acetaminophen as directed on package.** Check temperature every 15-30 minutes.

Watch the person's breathing. If it stops, see *Artificial Respiration*, p. 4

*If weather is very warm and person's skin does not feel cool and clammy,,covering will not be necessary.

**Do not give aspirin to a child with the flu.

14 Convulsion
(Including Epileptic Seizure)

Signs & Symptoms: *involuntary jerking of muscles/possible loss of bowel and bladder control/unconsciousness/cessation of breathing/gradual subsidence followed by semi-consciousness*

For any convulsions or seizures, obtain emergency assistance.

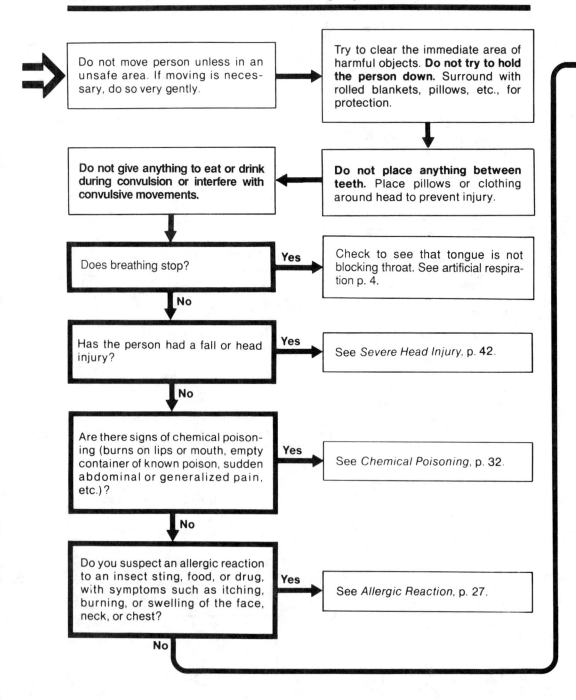

Do not move person unless in an unsafe area. If moving is necessary, do so very gently.

Try to clear the immediate area of harmful objects. **Do not try to hold the person down.** Surround with rolled blankets, pillows, etc., for protection.

Do not place anything between teeth. Place pillows or clothing around head to prevent injury.

Do not give anything to eat or drink during convulsion or interfere with convulsive movements.

Does breathing stop? — **Yes** → Check to see that tongue is not blocking throat. See artificial respiration p. 4.

No

Has the person had a fall or head injury? — **Yes** → See *Severe Head Injury*, p. 42.

No

Are there signs of chemical poisoning (burns on lips or mouth, empty container of known poison, sudden abdominal or generalized pain, etc.)? — **Yes** → See *Chemical Poisoning*, p. 32.

No

Do you suspect an allergic reaction to an insect sting, food, or drug, with symptoms such as itching, burning, or swelling of the face, neck, or chest? — **Yes** → See *Allergic Reaction*, p. 27.

No

Calm the person by talking while attending to the problem. Explain what you are doing. Try not to show anxiety; act with confidence. Your calm behavior can help to reassure the sick or injured person.

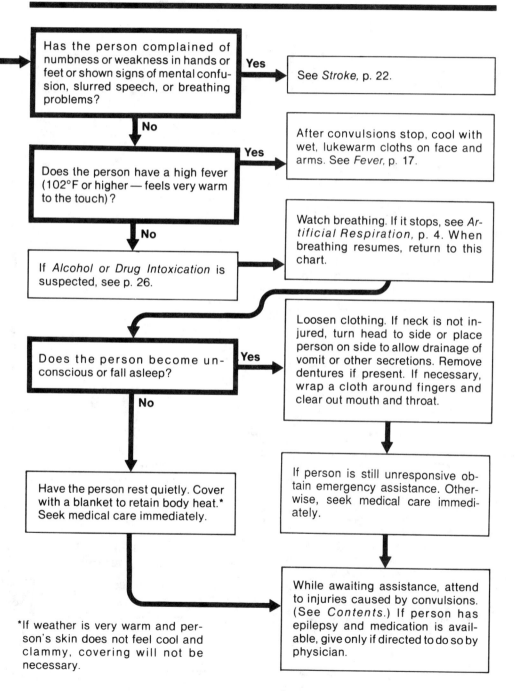

Has the person complained of numbness or weakness in hands or feet or shown signs of mental confusion, slurred speech, or breathing problems?

Yes → See *Stroke*, p. 22.

No

Does the person have a high fever (102°F or higher — feels very warm to the touch)?

Yes → After convulsions stop, cool with wet, lukewarm cloths on face and arms. See *Fever*, p. 17.

No

If *Alcohol or Drug Intoxication* is suspected, see p. 26.

Watch breathing. If it stops, see *Artificial Respiration*, p. 4. When breathing resumes, return to this chart.

Does the person become unconscious or fall asleep?

Yes → Loosen clothing. If neck is not injured, turn head to side or place person on side to allow drainage of vomit or other secretions. Remove dentures if present. If necessary, wrap a cloth around fingers and clear out mouth and throat.

No

Have the person rest quietly. Cover with a blanket to retain body heat.* Seek medical care immediately.

If person is still unresponsive obtain emergency assistance. Otherwise, seek medical care immediately.

*If weather is very warm and person's skin does not feel cool and clammy, covering will not be necessary.

While awaiting assistance, attend to injuries caused by convulsions. (See *Contents*.) If person has epilepsy and medication is available, give only if directed to do so by physician.

15 Croup Attack

Signs & Symptoms: *bark-like, ringing cough/ very difficult inhalation/possible difficulty exhaling/spasms or involuntary muscle contractions of the larynx (voice box)/tight, painful chest muscles/recent cold or upper respiratory infection/rapid pulse/possible fever/possible pale, bluish lips and nails*

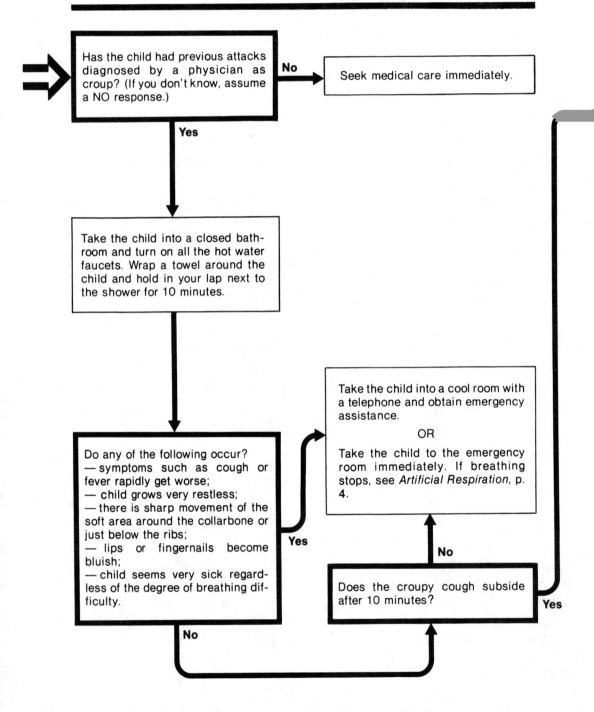

Has the child had previous attacks diagnosed by a physician as croup? (If you don't know, assume a NO response.)

No → Seek medical care immediately.

Yes

Take the child into a closed bathroom and turn on all the hot water faucets. Wrap a towel around the child and hold in your lap next to the shower for 10 minutes.

Do any of the following occur?
— symptoms such as cough or fever rapidly get worse;
— child grows very restless;
— there is sharp movement of the soft area around the collarbone or just below the ribs;
— lips or fingernails become bluish;
— child seems very sick regardless of the degree of breathing difficulty.

Yes →

Take the child into a cool room with a telephone and obtain emergency assistance.

OR

Take the child to the emergency room immediately. If breathing stops, see *Artificial Respiration*, p. 4.

No

Does the croupy cough subside after 10 minutes?

No ↑

Yes

No

Calm the person by talking while attending to the problem. Explain what you are doing. Try not to show anxiety; act with confidence. Your calm behavior can help to reassure the sick person.

If your child has a severe croup attack while traveling, seek medical care.

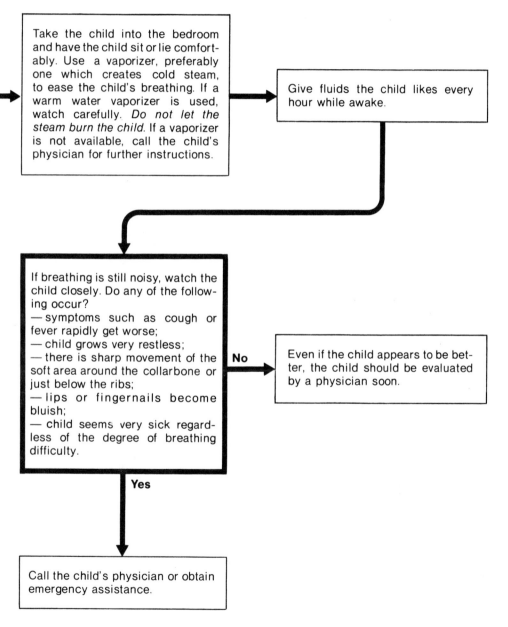

Take the child into the bedroom and have the child sit or lie comfortably. Use a vaporizer, preferably one which creates cold steam, to ease the child's breathing. If a warm water vaporizer is used, watch carefully. *Do not let the steam burn the child.* If a vaporizer is not available, call the child's physician for further instructions.

Give fluids the child likes every hour while awake.

If breathing is still noisy, watch the child closely. Do any of the following occur?
— symptoms such as cough or fever rapidly get worse;
— child grows very restless;
— there is sharp movement of the soft area around the collarbone or just below the ribs;
— lips or fingernails become bluish;
— child seems very sick regardless of the degree of breathing difficulty.

No

Even if the child appears to be better, the child should be evaluated by a physician soon.

Yes

Call the child's physician or obtain emergency assistance.

16 Diabetic Emergencies

Signs & Symptoms
diabetic coma (early warning): *flushed face/dry skin/ fruity breath odor/headache/thirst/drowsiness/ nausea/rapid pulse/rapid breathing/possible abdominal pain or vomiting*
insulin shock (early warning): *hunger/weakness/ shakiness/faintness/heavy sweating/blurred vision/ rapid pulse/cool and clammy skin/anxiety/restlessness/confusion.*

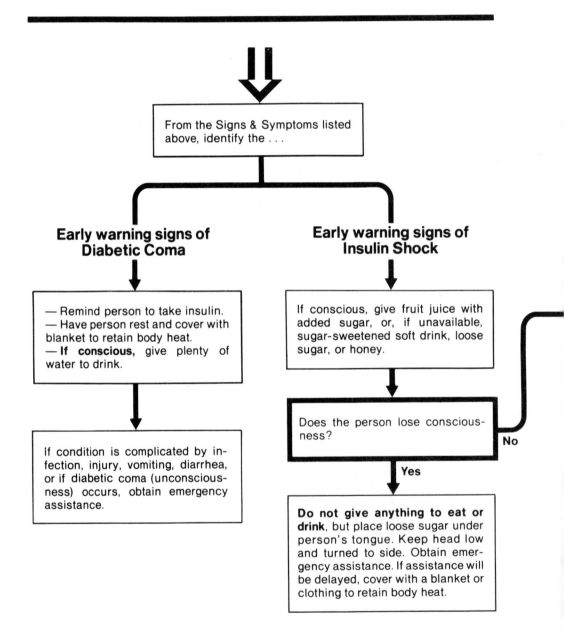

From the Signs & Symptoms listed above, identify the . . .

Early warning signs of Diabetic Coma

— Remind person to take insulin.
— Have person rest and cover with blanket to retain body heat.
— **If conscious,** give plenty of water to drink.

If condition is complicated by infection, injury, vomiting, diarrhea, or if diabetic coma (unconsciousness) occurs, obtain emergency assistance.

Early warning signs of Insulin Shock

If conscious, give fruit juice with added sugar, or, if unavailable, sugar-sweetened soft drink, loose sugar, or honey.

Does the person lose consciousness?

No

Yes

Do not give anything to eat or drink, but place loose sugar under person's tongue. Keep head low and turned to side. Obtain emergency assistance. If assistance will be delayed, cover with a blanket or clothing to retain body heat.

Calm the person by talking while attending to the problem. Explain what you are doing. Try not to show anxiety; act with confidence. Your calm behavior can help to reassure the sick person.

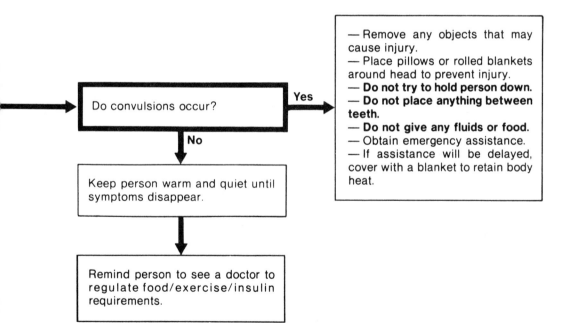

Do convulsions occur?

Yes

— Remove any objects that may cause injury.
— Place pillows or rolled blankets around head to prevent injury.
— **Do not try to hold person down.**
— **Do not place anything between teeth.**
— **Do not give any fluids or food.**
— Obtain emergency assistance.
— If assistance will be delayed, cover with a blanket to retain body heat.

No

Keep person warm and quiet until symptoms disappear.

Remind person to see a doctor to regulate food/exercise/insulin requirements.

17 Fever

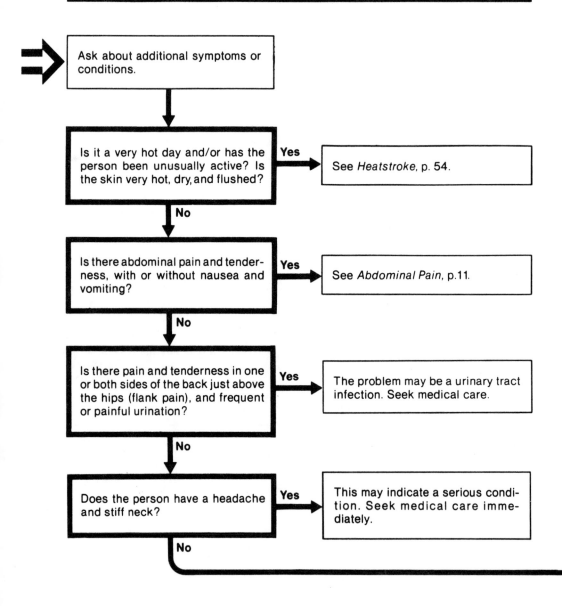

Ask about additional symptoms or conditions.

Is it a very hot day and/or has the person been unusually active? Is the skin very hot, dry, and flushed?

Yes → See *Heatstroke*, p. 54.

No

Is there abdominal pain and tenderness, with or without nausea and vomiting?

Yes → See *Abdominal Pain*, p.11.

No

Is there pain and tenderness in one or both sides of the back just above the hips (flank pain), and frequent or painful urination?

Yes → The problem may be a urinary tract infection. Seek medical care.

No

Does the person have a headache and stiff neck?

Yes → This may indicate a serious condition. Seek medical care immediately.

No

Calm the person by talking while attending to the problem. Explain what you are doing. Try not to show anxiety; act with confidence. Your calm behavior can help to reassure the sick person.

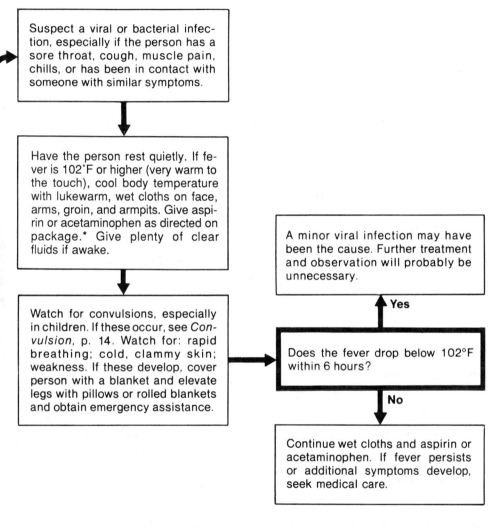

Suspect a viral or bacterial infection, especially if the person has a sore throat, cough, muscle pain, chills, or has been in contact with someone with similar symptoms.

Have the person rest quietly. If fever is 102°F or higher (very warm to the touch), cool body temperature with lukewarm, wet cloths on face, arms, groin, and armpits. Give aspirin or acetaminophen as directed on package.* Give plenty of clear fluids if awake.

A minor viral infection may have been the cause. Further treatment and observation will probably be unnecessary.

Watch for convulsions, especially in children. If these occur, see *Convulsion*, p. 14. Watch for: rapid breathing; cold, clammy skin; weakness. If these develop, cover person with a blanket and elevate legs with pillows or rolled blankets and obtain emergency assistance.

Does the fever drop below 102°F within 6 hours?

Yes

No

Continue wet cloths and aspirin or acetaminophen. If fever persists or additional symptoms develop, seek medical care.

*Do not give aspirin to a child with the flu.

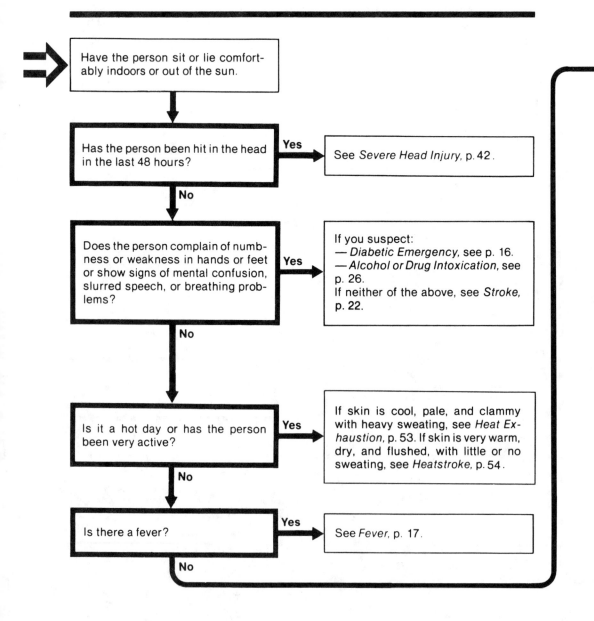

Have the person sit or lie comfortably indoors or out of the sun.

Has the person been hit in the head in the last 48 hours? — **Yes** → See *Severe Head Injury*, p. 42.

No

Does the person complain of numbness or weakness in hands or feet or show signs of mental confusion, slurred speech, or breathing problems? — **Yes** → If you suspect:
— *Diabetic Emergency*, see p. 16.
— *Alcohol or Drug Intoxication*, see p. 26.
If neither of the above, see *Stroke*, p. 22.

No

Is it a hot day or has the person been very active? — **Yes** → If skin is cool, pale, and clammy with heavy sweating, see *Heat Exhaustion*, p. 53. If skin is very warm, dry, and flushed, with little or no sweating, see *Heatstroke*, p. 54.

No

Is there a fever? — **Yes** → See *Fever*, p. 17.

No

Calm the person by talking while attending to the problem. Explain what you are doing. Try not to show anxiety; act with confidence. Your calm behavior can help to reassure the sick or injured person.

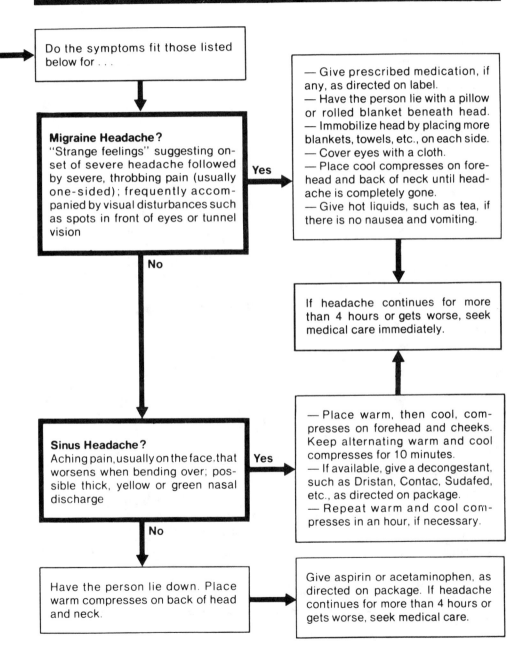

Do the symptoms fit those listed below for . . .

Migraine Headache?
"Strange feelings" suggesting onset of severe headache followed by severe, throbbing pain (usually one-sided); frequently accompanied by visual disturbances such as spots in front of eyes or tunnel vision

Yes →

— Give prescribed medication, if any, as directed on label.
— Have the person lie with a pillow or rolled blanket beneath head.
— Immobilize head by placing more blankets, towels, etc., on each side.
— Cover eyes with a cloth.
— Place cool compresses on forehead and back of neck until headache is completely gone.
— Give hot liquids, such as tea, if there is no nausea and vomiting.

If headache continues for more than 4 hours or gets worse, seek medical care immediately.

No ↓

Sinus Headache?
Aching pain, usually on the face, that worsens when bending over; possible thick, yellow or green nasal discharge

Yes →

— Place warm, then cool, compresses on forehead and cheeks. Keep alternating warm and cool compresses for 10 minutes.
— If available, give a decongestant, such as Dristan, Contac, Sudafed, etc., as directed on package.
— Repeat warm and cool compresses in an hour, if necessary.

No ↓

Have the person lie down. Place warm compresses on back of head and neck.

Give aspirin or acetaminophen, as directed on package. If headache continues for more than 4 hours or gets worse, seek medical care.

Internal
Bleeding

Possible Signs & Symptoms: *bloody or "coffee grounds" vomit/smoky or bloody urine/dark, bloody, or tar-like stools/pink or bloody sputum/ extreme paleness/weak or rapid pulse/cold, clammy skin/anxiety/thirst/rapid breathing/localized tenderness and swelling/rigid abdomen/ abdominal pain/unconsciousness*

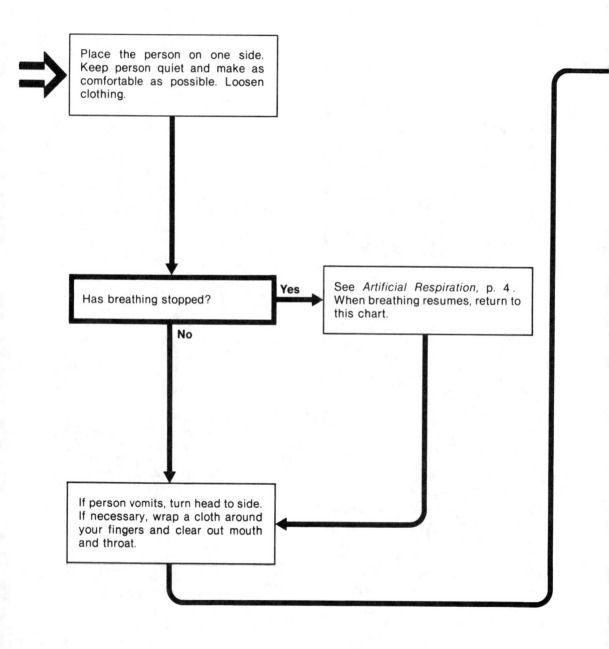

Place the person on one side. Keep person quiet and make as comfortable as possible. Loosen clothing.

Has breathing stopped?

Yes → See *Artificial Respiration,* p. 4. When breathing resumes, return to this chart.

No

If person vomits, turn head to side. If necessary, wrap a cloth around your fingers and clear out mouth and throat.

Calm the person by talking while attending to the problem. Explain what you are doing. Try not to show anxiety; act with confidence. Your calm behavior can help to reassure the sick person.

If there are two or more rescuers, one should obtain emergency assistance while the other is following the procedures outlined below.

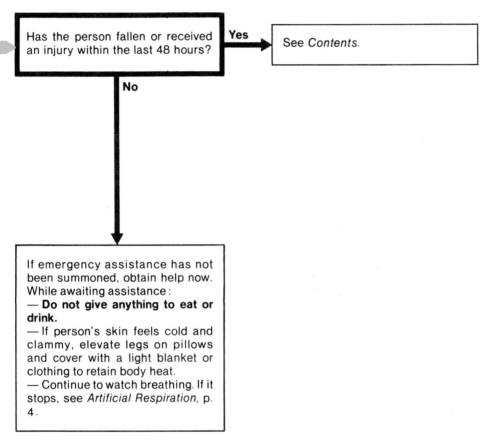

Has the person fallen or received an injury within the last 48 hours?

Yes → See *Contents*.

No

If emergency assistance has not been summoned, obtain help now. While awaiting assistance:
— **Do not give anything to eat or drink.**
— If person's skin feels cold and clammy, elevate legs on pillows and cover with a light blanket or clothing to retain body heat.
— Continue to watch breathing. If it stops, see *Artificial Respiration,* p. 4.

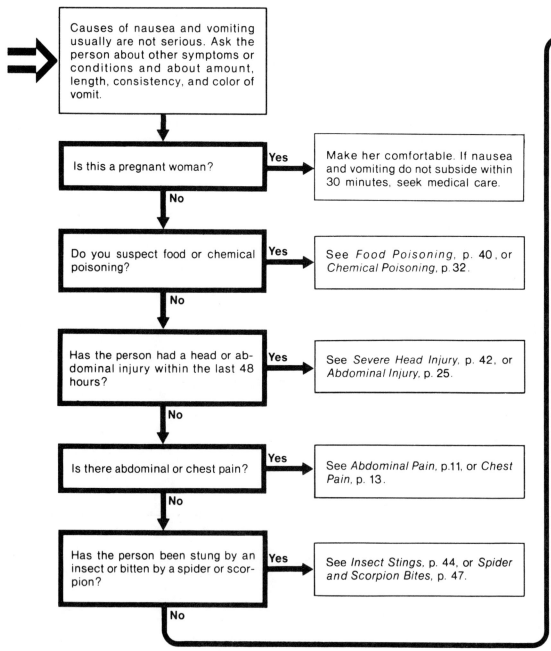

Causes of nausea and vomiting usually are not serious. Ask the person about other symptoms or conditions and about amount, length, consistency, and color of vomit.

Is this a pregnant woman?

Yes → Make her comfortable. If nausea and vomiting do not subside within 30 minutes, seek medical care.

No

Do you suspect food or chemical poisoning?

Yes → See *Food Poisoning*, p. 40, or *Chemical Poisoning*, p. 32.

No

Has the person had a head or abdominal injury within the last 48 hours?

Yes → See *Severe Head Injury*, p. 42, or *Abdominal Injury*, p. 25.

No

Is there abdominal or chest pain?

Yes → See *Abdominal Pain*, p.11, or *Chest Pain*, p. 13.

No

Has the person been stung by an insect or bitten by a spider or scorpion?

Yes → See *Insect Stings*, p. 44, or *Spider and Scorpion Bites*, p. 47.

No

Calm the person by talking while attending to the problem. Explain what you are doing. Try not to show anxiety; act with confidence. Your calm behavior can help to reassure the sick or injured person.

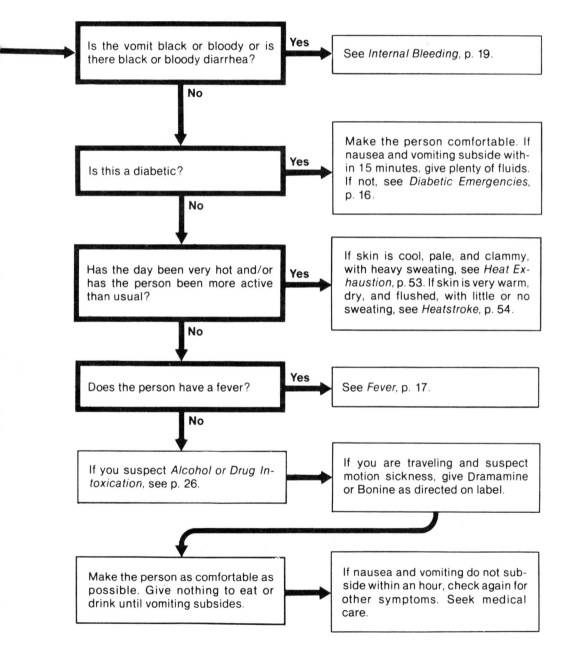

Is the vomit black or bloody or is there black or bloody diarrhea?

Yes → See *Internal Bleeding*, p. 19.

No

Is this a diabetic?

Yes → Make the person comfortable. If nausea and vomiting subside within 15 minutes, give plenty of fluids. If not, see *Diabetic Emergencies*, p. 16.

No

Has the day been very hot and/or has the person been more active than usual?

Yes → If skin is cool, pale, and clammy, with heavy sweating, see *Heat Exhaustion*, p. 53. If skin is very warm, dry, and flushed, with little or no sweating, see *Heatstroke*, p. 54.

No

Does the person have a fever?

Yes → See *Fever*, p. 17.

No

If you suspect *Alcohol or Drug Intoxication*, see p. 26.

→ If you are traveling and suspect motion sickness, give Dramamine or Bonine as directed on label.

Make the person as comfortable as possible. Give nothing to eat or drink until vomiting subsides.

→ If nausea and vomiting do not subside within an hour, check again for other symptoms. Seek medical care.

21Nosebleed

Do not stuff cotton or tissues into the nose.

If person fell or received a head injury, see *Severe Head Injury,* **p. 42.**

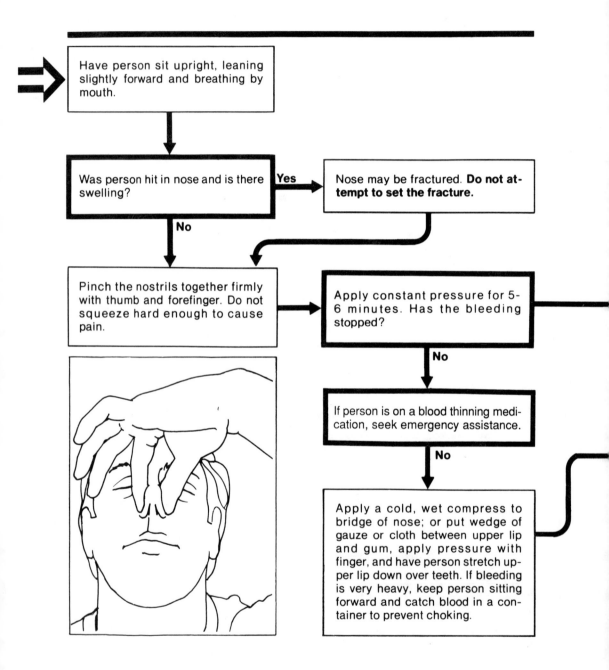

Have person sit upright, leaning slightly forward and breathing by mouth.

Was person hit in nose and is there swelling? **Yes** → Nose may be fractured. **Do not attempt to set the fracture.**

No

Pinch the nostrils together firmly with thumb and forefinger. Do not squeeze hard enough to cause pain.

Apply constant pressure for 5-6 minutes. Has the bleeding stopped?

No

If person is on a blood thinning medication, seek emergency assistance.

No

Apply a cold, wet compress to bridge of nose; or put wedge of gauze or cloth between upper lip and gum, apply pressure with finger, and have person stretch upper lip down over teeth. If bleeding is very heavy, keep person sitting forward and catch blood in a container to prevent choking.

Calm the person by talking while attending to the problem. Explain what you are doing. Try not to show anxiety; act with confidence. Your calm behavior can help to reassure the sick or injured person.

If the injury was the result of a vehicular or job-related accident, the person should be examined by a physician for possible additional injuries or complications.

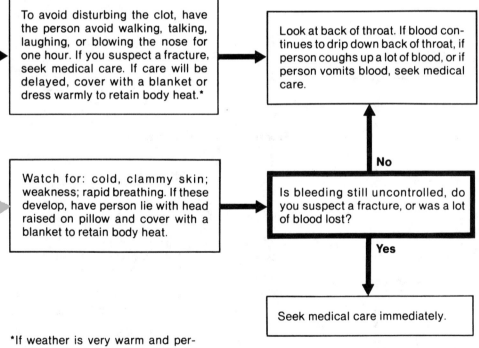

To avoid disturbing the clot, have the person avoid walking, talking, laughing, or blowing the nose for one hour. If you suspect a fracture, seek medical care. If care will be delayed, cover with a blanket or dress warmly to retain body heat.*

Look at back of throat. If blood continues to drip down back of throat, if person coughs up a lot of blood, or if person vomits blood, seek medical care.

Watch for: cold, clammy skin; weakness; rapid breathing. If these develop, have person lie with head raised on pillow and cover with a blanket to retain body heat.

No

Is bleeding still uncontrolled, do you suspect a fracture, or was a lot of blood lost?

Yes

Seek medical care immediately.

*If weather is very warm and person's skin does not feel cool and clammy, covering will not be necessary.

22 Stroke

Possible Signs & Symptoms: *stiffness or paralysis of facial muscles, extremities, either side of body/breathing or swallowing difficulty/confusion/dizziness/loss of bladder or bowel control/pupils unequal in size/headache/blurred vision/slurred speech or inability to speak/convulsions/unconsciousness/coma*

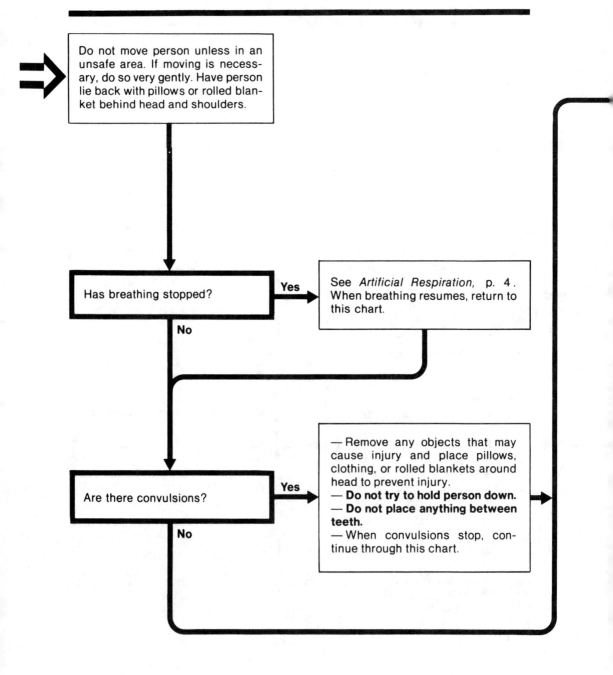

Do not move person unless in an unsafe area. If moving is necessary, do so very gently. Have person lie back with pillows or rolled blanket behind head and shoulders.

Has breathing stopped?

Yes → See *Artificial Respiration*, p. 4. When breathing resumes, return to this chart.

No

Are there convulsions?

Yes →
— Remove any objects that may cause injury and place pillows, clothing, or rolled blankets around head to prevent injury.
— **Do not try to hold person down.**
— **Do not place anything between teeth.**
— When convulsions stop, continue through this chart.

No

Calm the person by talking while attending to the problem. Explain what you are doing. Try not to show anxiety; act with confidence. Your calm behavior can help to reassure the sick person.

If there are two or more rescuers, one should obtain emergency assistance while the other is following the procedures outlined below.

If the person is unconscious or appears to be choking, turn head to side to allow drainage of secretions. Remove dentures if loose. If necessary, wrap a cloth around your fingers and clear out mouth and throat. **Do not give anything to eat or drink.**

If you do *not* suspect a fracture, gently straighten any twisted or paralyzed limb(s) to maintain proper circulation.

If emergency assistance has not been summoned, obtain help now. While awaiting assistance:
— Continue to check breathing. If it stops, see *Artificial Respiration,* p. 4.
— Watch for shock: cold, clammy skin; rapid breathing; weakness. If these develop, cover with blanket or clothing to retain body heat.

23 Toothache or Lost or Broken Tooth

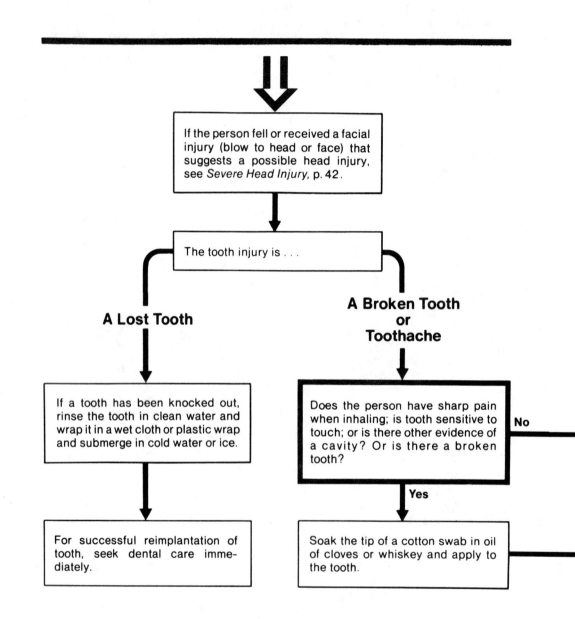

If the person fell or received a facial injury (blow to head or face) that suggests a possible head injury, see *Severe Head Injury*, p. 42.

The tooth injury is . . .

A Lost Tooth

A Broken Tooth or Toothache

If a tooth has been knocked out, rinse the tooth in clean water and wrap it in a wet cloth or plastic wrap and submerge in cold water or ice.

Does the person have sharp pain when inhaling; is tooth sensitive to touch; or is there other evidence of a cavity? Or is there a broken tooth?

No

Yes

For successful reimplantation of tooth, seek dental care immediately.

Soak the tip of a cotton swab in oil of cloves or whiskey and apply to the tooth.

Calm the person by talking while attending to the problem. Explain what you are doing. Try not to show anxiety; act with confidence. Your calm behavior can help to reassure the injured person.

If injury was the result of a vehicular or job-related accident, the person should be examined by a physician for possible additional injuries or complications.

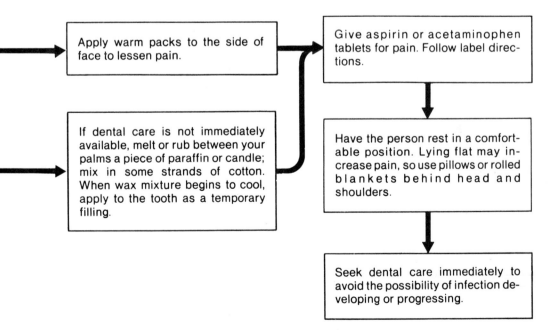

Apply warm packs to the side of face to lessen pain.

Give aspirin or acetaminophen tablets for pain. Follow label directions.

If dental care is not immediately available, melt or rub between your palms a piece of paraffin or candle; mix in some strands of cotton. When wax mixture begins to cool, apply to the tooth as a temporary filling.

Have the person rest in a comfortable position. Lying flat may increase pain, so use pillows or rolled blankets behind head and shoulders.

Seek dental care immediately to avoid the possibility of infection developing or progressing.

24 Unconsciousness

Shout for help even if you think you are alone. If there are two or more rescuers, one should obtain emergency assistance while the other is following the procedures outlined below.

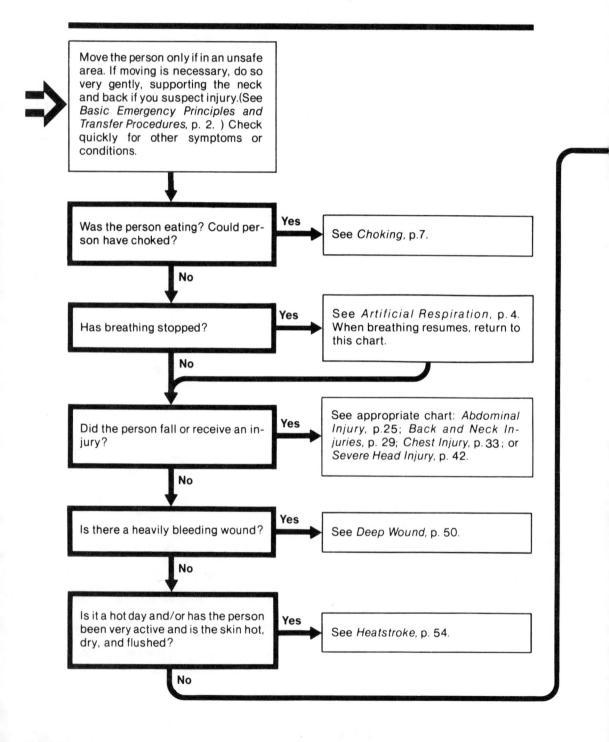

Move the person only if in an unsafe area. If moving is necessary, do so very gently, supporting the neck and back if you suspect injury.(See *Basic Emergency Principles and Transfer Procedures*, p. 2.) Check quickly for other symptoms or conditions.

Was the person eating? Could person have choked?

Yes → See *Choking*, p.7.

No

Has breathing stopped?

Yes → See *Artificial Respiration*, p. 4. When breathing resumes, return to this chart.

No

Did the person fall or receive an injury?

Yes → See appropriate chart: *Abdominal Injury*, p.25; *Back and Neck Injuries*, p. 29; *Chest Injury*, p. 33; or *Severe Head Injury*, p. 42.

No

Is there a heavily bleeding wound?

Yes → See *Deep Wound*, p. 50.

No

Is it a hot day and/or has the person been very active and is the skin hot, dry, and flushed?

Yes → See *Heatstroke*, p. 54.

No

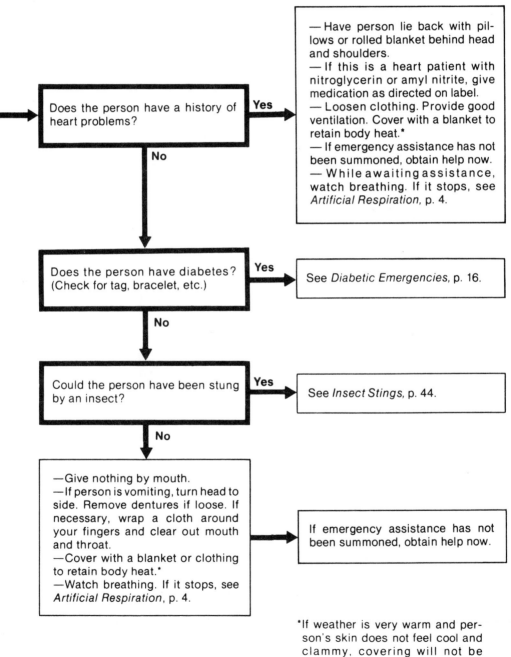

Does the person have a history of heart problems?

Yes →

— Have person lie back with pillows or rolled blanket behind head and shoulders.
— If this is a heart patient with nitroglycerin or amyl nitrite, give medication as directed on label.
— Loosen clothing. Provide good ventilation. Cover with a blanket to retain body heat.*
— If emergency assistance has not been summoned, obtain help now.
— While awaiting assistance, watch breathing. If it stops, see *Artificial Respiration*, p. 4.

No ↓

Does the person have diabetes? (Check for tag, bracelet, etc.)

Yes →

See *Diabetic Emergencies*, p. 16.

No ↓

Could the person have been stung by an insect?

Yes →

See *Insect Stings*, p. 44.

No ↓

—Give nothing by mouth.
—If person is vomiting, turn head to side. Remove dentures if loose. If necessary, wrap a cloth around your fingers and clear out mouth and throat.
—Cover with a blanket or clothing to retain body heat.*
—Watch breathing. If it stops, see *Artificial Respiration*, p. 4.

→

If emergency assistance has not been summoned, obtain help now.

*If weather is very warm and person's skin does not feel cool and clammy, covering will not be necessary.

25 Abdominal Injury

Signs & Symptoms
Internal bleeding: swelling/discoloration/ severe pain/cold, clammy skin/restlessness/ thirst/vomiting or coughing blood/blood in urine or feces
Hernia: pain, swelling, or discoloration in groin or scrotum

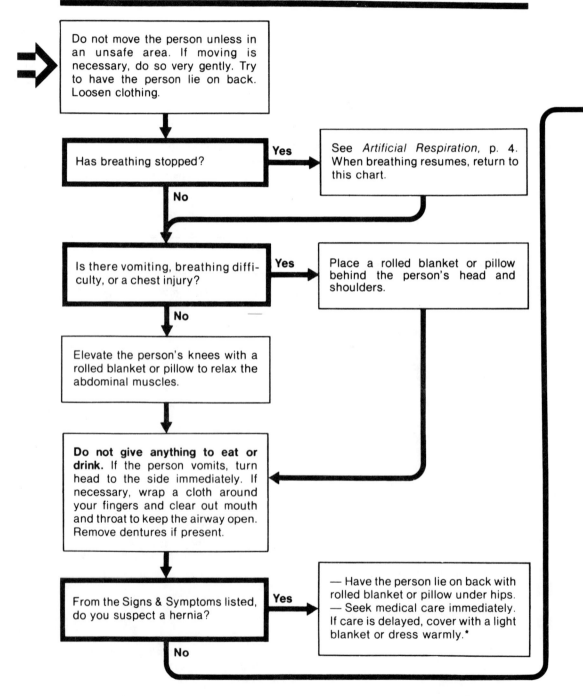

Do not move the person unless in an unsafe area. If moving is necessary, do so very gently. Try to have the person lie on back. Loosen clothing.

Has breathing stopped?

Yes → See *Artificial Respiration,* p. 4. When breathing resumes, return to this chart.

No

Is there vomiting, breathing difficulty, or a chest injury?

Yes → Place a rolled blanket or pillow behind the person's head and shoulders.

No

Elevate the person's knees with a rolled blanket or pillow to relax the abdominal muscles.

Do not give anything to eat or drink. If the person vomits, turn head to the side immediately. If necessary, wrap a cloth around your fingers and clear out mouth and throat to keep the airway open. Remove dentures if present.

From the Signs & Symptoms listed, do you suspect a hernia?

Yes → — Have the person lie on back with rolled blanket or pillow under hips.
— Seek medical care immediately. If care is delayed, cover with a light blanket or dress warmly.*

No

Calm the person by talking while attending to the problem. Explain what you are doing. Try not to show anxiety; act with confidence. Your calm behavior can help to reassure the injured person.

If there was a severe blow to the head or a fall, or if person is unconscious, assume neck injury and do not move.

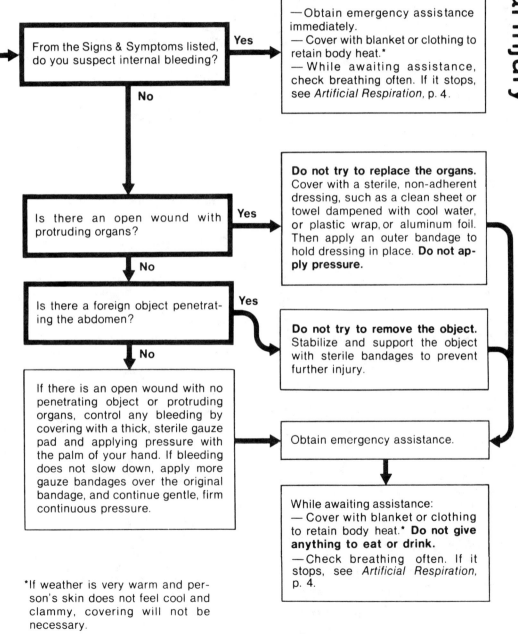

From the Signs & Symptoms listed, do you suspect internal bleeding?

Yes → —Obtain emergency assistance immediately.
— Cover with blanket or clothing to retain body heat.*
— While awaiting assistance, check breathing often. If it stops, see *Artificial Respiration*, p. 4.

No

Is there an open wound with protruding organs?

Yes → **Do not try to replace the organs.** Cover with a sterile, non-adherent dressing, such as a clean sheet or towel dampened with cool water, or plastic wrap, or aluminum foil. Then apply an outer bandage to hold dressing in place. **Do not apply pressure.**

No

Is there a foreign object penetrating the abdomen?

Yes → **Do not try to remove the object.** Stabilize and support the object with sterile bandages to prevent further injury.

No

If there is an open wound with no penetrating object or protruding organs, control any bleeding by covering with a thick, sterile gauze pad and applying pressure with the palm of your hand. If bleeding does not slow down, apply more gauze bandages over the original bandage, and continue gentle, firm continuous pressure.

→ Obtain emergency assistance.

While awaiting assistance:
— Cover with blanket or clothing to retain body heat.* **Do not give anything to eat or drink.**
—Check breathing often. If it stops, see *Artificial Respiration*, p. 4.

*If weather is very warm and person's skin does not feel cool and clammy, covering will not be necessary.

26 Alcohol or Drug Intoxication

Possible Signs & Symptoms: *restlessness/ confusion/slurred speech/flushed skin/hallucin- ations/pinpoint or dilated pupils/muscular twitching/tremors/nausea and vomiting/ drowsiness/shallow breathing/cold sweat/ dizziness/irritability/fear/depression/violent or ag- gressive behavior/convulsions/unconscious- ness. Symptoms will vary with different drugs.* For *Allergic Reaction,* see p. 27.

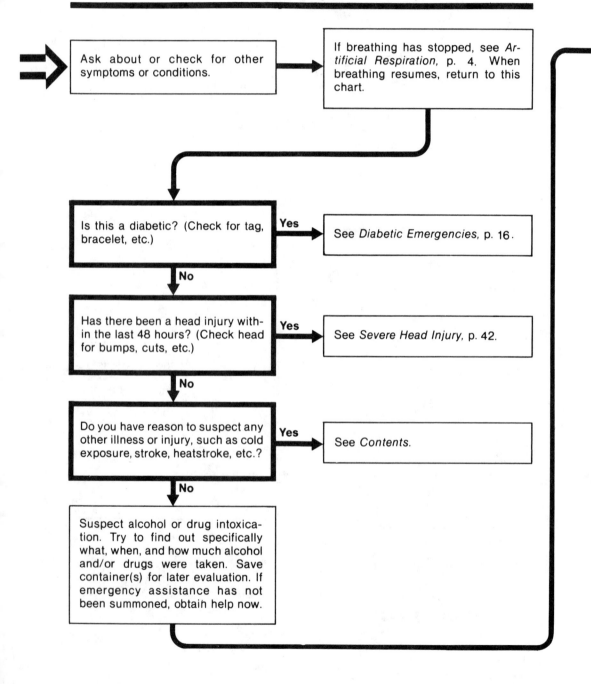

Ask about or check for other symptoms or conditions.

If breathing has stopped, see *Artificial Respiration,* p. 4. When breathing resumes, return to this chart.

Is this a diabetic? (Check for tag, bracelet, etc.)

Yes → See *Diabetic Emergencies,* p. 16.

No

Has there been a head injury with- in the last 48 hours? (Check head for bumps, cuts, etc.)

Yes → See *Severe Head Injury,* p. 42.

No

Do you have reason to suspect any other illness or injury, such as cold exposure, stroke, heatstroke, etc.?

Yes → See *Contents.*

No

Suspect alcohol or drug intoxica- tion. Try to find out specifically what, when, and how much alcohol and/or drugs were taken. Save container(s) for later evaluation. If emergency assistance has not been summoned, obtain help now.

Calm the person by talking while attending to the problem. Explain what you are doing. Try not to show anxiety; act with confidence. Your calm behavior can help to reassure the sick person.

If there are two or more rescuers, one should obtain emergency assistance while the other is following the procedures outlined below.

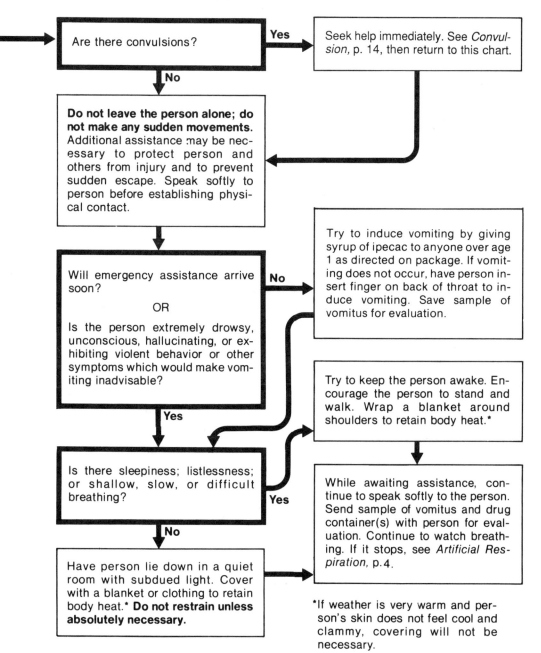

Are there convulsions? — **Yes** → Seek help immediately. See *Convulsion*, p. 14, then return to this chart.

No ↓

Do not leave the person alone; do not make any sudden movements. Additional assistance may be necessary to protect person and others from injury and to prevent sudden escape. Speak softly to person before establishing physical contact.

Will emergency assistance arrive soon?

OR

Is the person extremely drowsy, unconscious, hallucinating, or exhibiting violent behavior or other symptoms which would make vomiting inadvisable? — **No** → Try to induce vomiting by giving syrup of ipecac to anyone over age 1 as directed on package. If vomiting does not occur, have person insert finger on back of throat to induce vomiting. Save sample of vomitus for evaluation.

Yes ↓

Is there sleepiness; listlessness; or shallow, slow, or difficult breathing? — **Yes** → Try to keep the person awake. Encourage the person to stand and walk. Wrap a blanket around shoulders to retain body heat.*

→ While awaiting assistance, continue to speak softly to the person. Send sample of vomitus and drug container(s) with person for evaluation. Continue to watch breathing. If it stops, see *Artificial Respiration*, p.4.

No ↓

Have person lie down in a quiet room with subdued light. Cover with a blanket or clothing to retain body heat.* **Do not restrain unless absolutely necessary.**

*If weather is very warm and person's skin does not feel cool and clammy, covering will not be necessary.

27 Allergic Reaction

For drug intoxication with no allergic reaction, see *Alcohol or Drug Intoxication*, p. 26.

Possible Signs & Symptoms: *itching, flushing, or burning, especially near face or chest/hives/ edema, particularly of face, neck, tongue, and lips/tightness or pain in chest or throat/coughing or wheezing/breathing difficulty/pale skin/dizziness/convulsions/unconsciousness/coma*

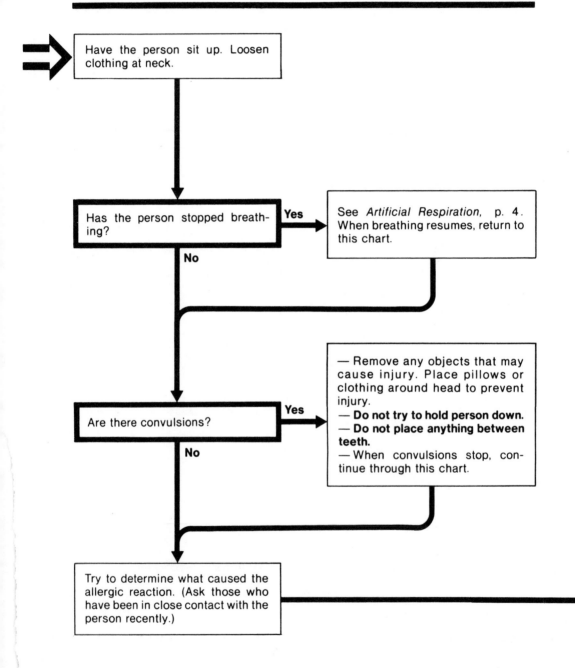

Have the person sit up. Loosen clothing at neck.

Has the person stopped breathing?

Yes → See *Artificial Respiration*, p. 4. When breathing resumes, return to this chart.

No

Are there convulsions?

Yes → — Remove any objects that may cause injury. Place pillows or clothing around head to prevent injury.
— **Do not try to hold person down.**
— **Do not place anything between teeth.**
— When convulsions stop, continue through this chart.

No

Try to determine what caused the allergic reaction. (Ask those who have been in close contact with the person recently.)

Calm the person by talking while attending to the problem. Explain what you are doing. Try not to show anxiety; act with confidence. Your calm behavior can help to reassure the sick person.

If there are two or more rescuers, one should obtain emergency assistance while the other is following the procedures outlined below.

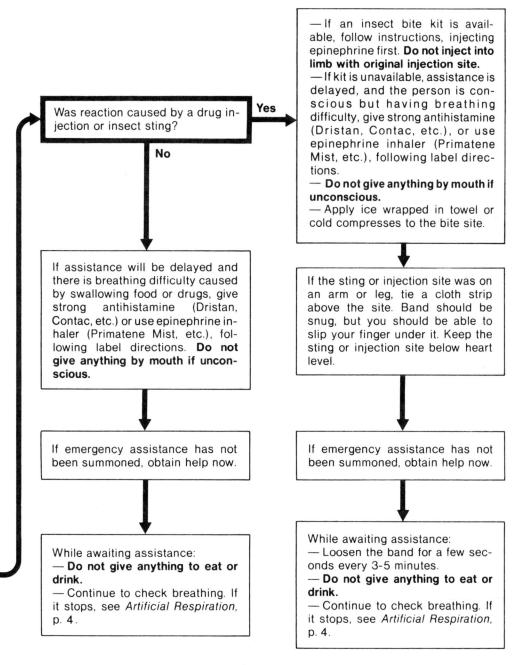

Was reaction caused by a drug injection or insect sting?

Yes

No

—If an insect bite kit is available, follow instructions, injecting epinephrine first. **Do not inject into limb with original injection site.**
—If kit is unavailable, assistance is delayed, and the person is conscious but having breathing difficulty, give strong antihistamine (Dristan, Contac, etc.), or use epinephrine inhaler (Primatene Mist, etc.), following label directions.
— **Do not give anything by mouth if unconscious.**
— Apply ice wrapped in towel or cold compresses to the bite site.

If assistance will be delayed and there is breathing difficulty caused by swallowing food or drugs, give strong antihistamine (Dristan, Contac, etc.) or use epinephrine inhaler (Primatene Mist, etc.), following label directions. **Do not give anything by mouth if unconscious.**

If the sting or injection site was on an arm or leg, tie a cloth strip above the site. Band should be snug, but you should be able to slip your finger under it. Keep the sting or injection site below heart level.

If emergency assistance has not been summoned, obtain help now.

If emergency assistance has not been summoned, obtain help now.

While awaiting assistance:
— **Do not give anything to eat or drink.**
— Continue to check breathing. If it stops, see *Artificial Respiration*, p. 4.

While awaiting assistance:
— Loosen the band for a few seconds every 3-5 minutes.
— **Do not give anything to eat or drink.**
— Continue to check breathing. If it stops, see *Artificial Respiration*, p. 4.

28 Animal and Human Bites

If there are two or more rescuers, one should attend to the person, while the other tries to trap animal to check later for rabies. **Be careful not to get bitten.** If capturing the animal is not possible, note behavior for later evaluation. (All animal and human bites must be reported to local police and/or health officer.)

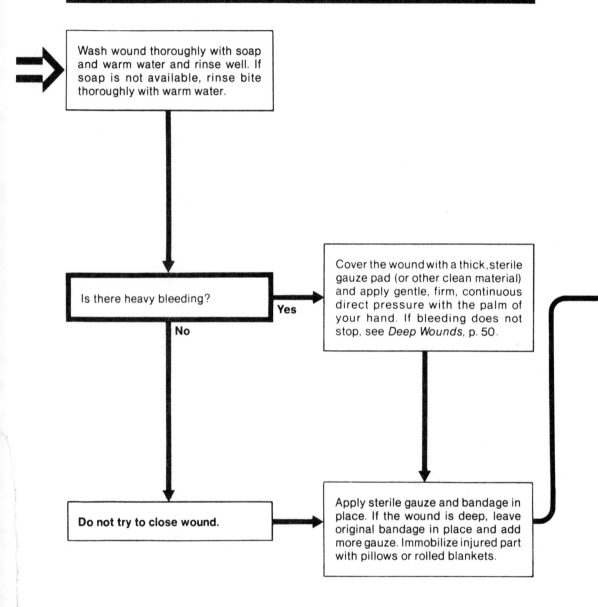

Wash wound thoroughly with soap and warm water and rinse well. If soap is not available, rinse bite thoroughly with warm water.

Is there heavy bleeding?

Yes

No

Cover the wound with a thick, sterile gauze pad (or other clean material) and apply gentle, firm, continuous direct pressure with the palm of your hand. If bleeding does not stop, see *Deep Wounds*, p. 50.

Do not try to close wound.

Apply sterile gauze and bandage in place. If the wound is deep, leave original bandage in place and add more gauze. Immobilize injured part with pillows or rolled blankets.

Calm the person by talking while attending to the problem. Explain what you are doing. Try not to show anxiety; act with confidence. Your calm behavior can help to reassure the injured person.

If the wounds are severe, check breathing. If it stops, see *Artificial Respiration*, p.4.

Watch for: cold, clammy skin; weakness; rapid breathing. If these develop, cover with a blanket or clothing to retain body heat. If no heart problems or head injuries are present, elevate the legs on a pillow or rolled blanket.

Make person comfortable. Seek medical care. Person may require tetanus immunization and possibly rabies vaccination.

29 Back & Neck Injuries

Do not move someone with severe back or neck injuries unless absolutely necessary.

Signs & Symptoms: *Severe pain and tenderness at site of injury/possible deformity of injured area/possible paralysis of one or more limbs/pain on movement*

With any severe fall or other severe trauma injuring the back, assume fractures of both neck and back. If person is unconscious from a direct blow to the head or a fall, assume neck fracture.

Secure the neck very carefully with a collar (use rolled towel). Be sure to keep the head straight; do not raise or lower chin or turn head.

If breathing has stopped, gently roll person onto back, keeping neck and back as straight as possible. See *Artificial Respiration,* p. 4. When breathing resumes, return to this chart.

Leave in present position. Immobilize by placing pillows or rolled blankets around entire body. Cover with a blanket to retain body heat.* Obtain emergency assistance. Check breathing often. If it stops, see *Artificial Respiration,* p. 4.

Yes ← Is the person lying in a safe area?

No

Are there two or more rescuers? AND Is a spineboard or makeshift board (mattress board, ironing board, door, leaf from a table, etc.) available?

No

Yes ←

— Place a spineboard or makeshift board beside the person.
— *Rescuers:* Position yourselves as shown below, then grasp with both hands the seams on the side of person's clothing nearest board.
— *Rescuer at the head:* Direct the turning of the body simultaneously and slowly, rolling the person toward the rescuers, keeping the body and head straight.

— The middle rescuer slides the board underneath the person with one arm, while the others hold the person in place. Then roll the person back simultaneously and slowly, keeping the body and head straight.
— Immobilize the person's head with pillows, towels, etc., without lifting or moving the head.
— Secure the person to the board with belts, ties, straps, rope, etc.
— Then lift the board slowly and simultaneously and walk carefully to safety.
— Obtain emergency assistance.
— While waiting for help, make person comfortable and cover with a blanket to retain body heat.* Check breathing often. If it stops, see *Artificial Respiration,* p. 4.

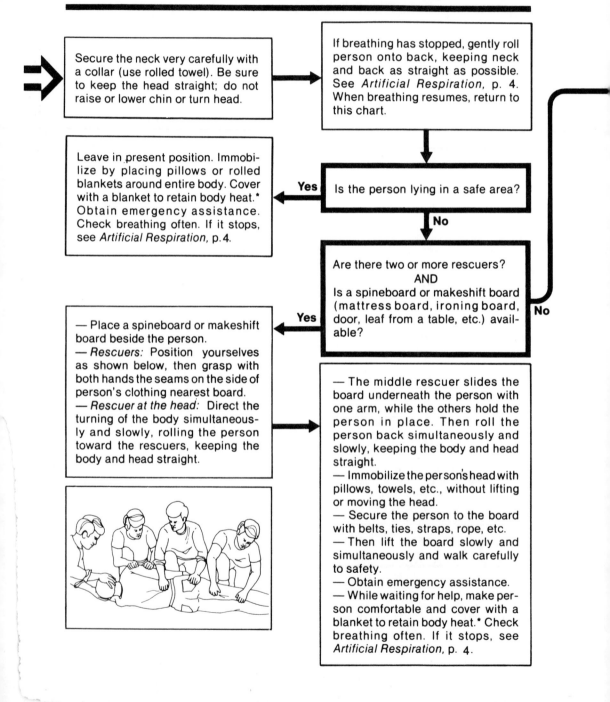

Calm the person by talking while attending to the problem. Explain what you are doing. Try not to show anxiety; act with confidence. Your calm behavior can help to reassure the injured person.

Place your hands under the armpits and cradle the neck and head with your forearms. Gently pull to safety, keeping body straight. Cover with a blanket or clothing to retain body heat.*

Immobilize by placing pillows or rolled blankets around entire body. Obtain emergency assistance. While awaiting assistance, watch breathing. If it stops, see *Artificial Respiration,* p. 4. Attend to other injuries. (See *Contents.*)

*If weather is very warm and person's skin does not feel cool and clammy, covering will not be necessary.

30 Bruise

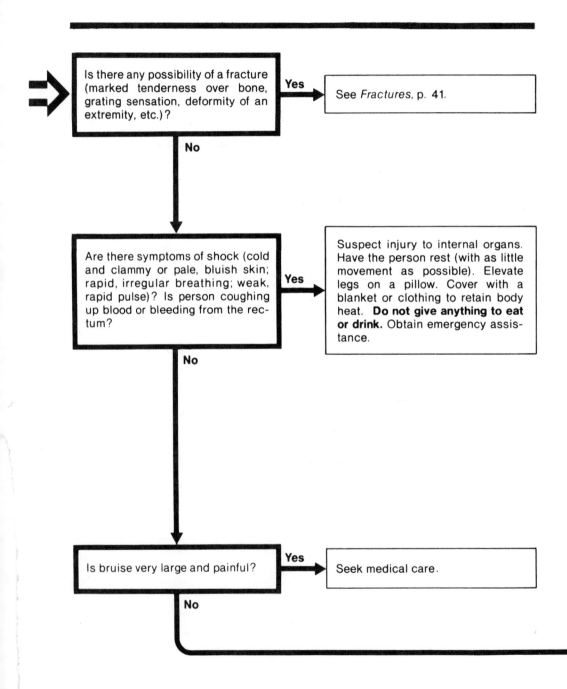

Signs & Symptoms: *pain and tenderness at site of injury/black and blue appearance of skin (may be delayed, with redness appearing first)*

For severe bruise on head, see *Severe Head Injury*, p. 42.

Is there any possibility of a fracture (marked tenderness over bone, grating sensation, deformity of an extremity, etc.)?

Yes → See *Fractures*, p. 41.

No

Are there symptoms of shock (cold and clammy or pale, bluish skin; rapid, irregular breathing; weak, rapid pulse)? Is person coughing up blood or bleeding from the rectum?

Yes → Suspect injury to internal organs. Have the person rest (with as little movement as possible). Elevate legs on a pillow. Cover with a blanket or clothing to retain body heat. **Do not give anything to eat or drink.** Obtain emergency assistance.

No

Is bruise very large and painful?

Yes → Seek medical care.

No

Calm the person by talking while attending to the problem. Explain what you are doing. Try not to show anxiety; act with confidence. Your calm behavior can help to reassure the injured person.

If injury was the result of a vehicular or job-related accident, the person should be examined by a physician for possible additional injuries or complications.

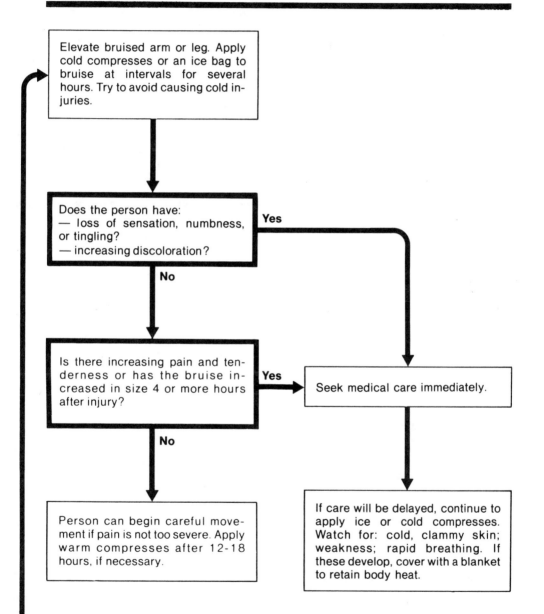

31 Burns

(Including Lightning, Electric Shock, Chemical Burns, and Sunburn)

First Degree: redness of skin/pain, perhaps with mild swelling. First degree burns involving over 10% of the body should be considered third degree.

Second Degree: deep reddening of skin/skin has glossy appearance from leaking fluid (plasma)/possible loss of some skin/blisters. Second degree burns involving over 10% of the body should be considered third degree.

Third Degree: loss of all skin layers/painless/possible charring of skin edges/involving more than a very small area.

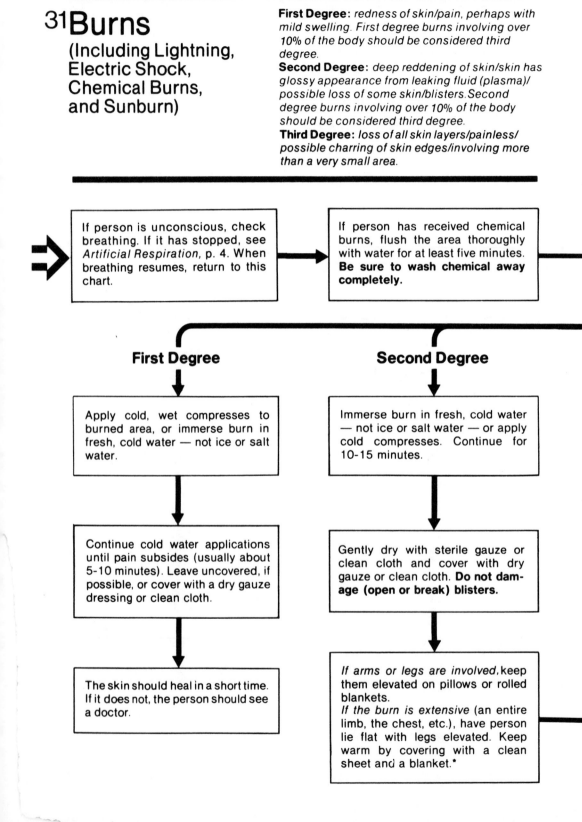

If person is unconscious, check breathing. If it has stopped, see *Artificial Respiration*, p. 4. When breathing resumes, return to this chart.

If person has received chemical burns, flush the area thoroughly with water for at least five minutes. **Be sure to wash chemical away completely.**

First Degree

Apply cold, wet compresses to burned area, or immerse burn in fresh, cold water — not ice or salt water.

Continue cold water applications until pain subsides (usually about 5-10 minutes). Leave uncovered, if possible, or cover with a dry gauze dressing or clean cloth.

The skin should heal in a short time. If it does not, the person should see a doctor.

Second Degree

Immerse burn in fresh, cold water — not ice or salt water — or apply cold compresses. Continue for 10-15 minutes.

Gently dry with sterile gauze or clean cloth and cover with dry gauze or clean cloth. **Do not damage (open or break) blisters.**

If arms or legs are involved, keep them elevated on pillows or rolled blankets.
If the burn is extensive (an entire limb, the chest, etc.), have person lie flat with legs elevated. Keep warm by covering with a clean sheet and a blanket.*

In cases of electric shock, if person is still touching electrical source, do not touch either the person or the source. First, turn off master electrical switch or pull appliance plug. If caused by fallen electrical wire, do not try to move the wire away. Instead, obtain emergency assistance (i.e., police, fire departments, etc.)

Calm the person by talking while attending to the problem. Explain what you are doing. Try not to show anxiety; act with confidence. Your calm behavior can help to reassure the injured person.

Gently move person to a safe, warm, sheltered area. Remove clothing and jewelry from burn area (cut it away, if necessary). If clothing sticks to the burn, do not try to remove it.

Based on the Signs & Symptoms listed above, determine whether the burn is first, second, or third degree. If you're in doubt, choose the more serious classification.

Third Degree

Cover burn lightly with sterile gauze or clean cloth. (Do not use material that can leave lint in burn.) **Unless this is a chemical burn, do not use wet compresses and do not immerse burn in water.**

Have person lie flat with legs elevated on pillows or rolled blanket to prevent shock .

No ← Is face or head burned?

Yes

If arms are burned, keep them elevated as well. Cover person with a clean cloth and a blanket.*

Have person sit up. Watch closely for possible breathing problems. If breathing stops, see *Artificial Respiration*, p. 4, then return to this chart.

— Obtain emergency assistance.
— While awaiting assistance, check breathing often. If it stops, see *Artificial Respiration*, p. 4.

*If weather is very warm and person's skin does not feel cool and clammy, covering will not be necessary.

32 Chemical Poisoning

Signs & Symptoms: *an empty container of known poison/sudden onset of abdominal or generalized pain/nausea and vomiting may or may not be present/burns on lips and mouth/distinctive breath odor/stupor or unconsciousness. Symptoms will vary depending on type of poison.*

Contact poison control immediately even if you only suspect poisoning.

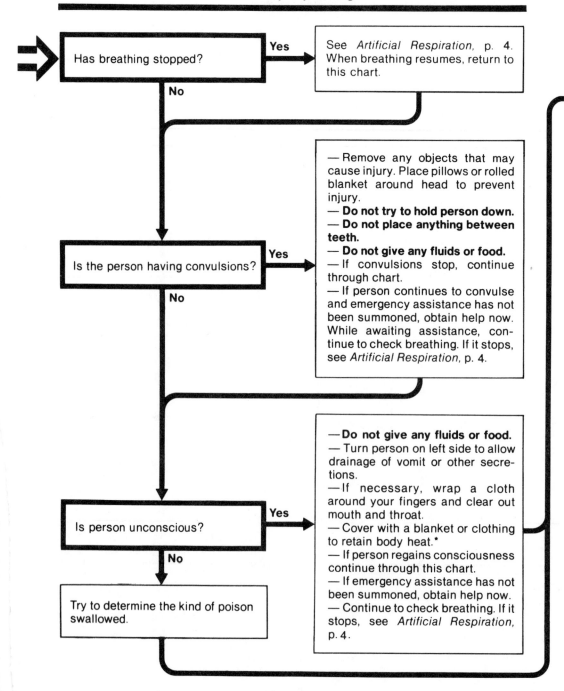

Has breathing stopped? — **Yes** → See *Artificial Respiration,* p. 4. When breathing resumes, return to this chart.

No

Is the person having convulsions? — **Yes** →
— Remove any objects that may cause injury. Place pillows or rolled blanket around head to prevent injury.
— **Do not try to hold person down.**
— **Do not place anything between teeth.**
— **Do not give any fluids or food.**
— If convulsions stop, continue through chart.
— If person continues to convulse and emergency assistance has not been summoned, obtain help now. While awaiting assistance, continue to check breathing. If it stops, see *Artificial Respiration,* p. 4.

No

Is person unconscious? — **Yes** →
— **Do not give any fluids or food.**
— Turn person on left side to allow drainage of vomit or other secretions.
— If necessary, wrap a cloth around your fingers and clear out mouth and throat.
— Cover with a blanket or clothing to retain body heat.*
— If person regains consciousness continue through this chart.
— If emergency assistance has not been summoned, obtain help now.
— Continue to check breathing. If it stops, see *Artificial Respiration,* p. 4.

No

Try to determine the kind of poison swallowed.

Calm the person by talking while attending to the problem. Explain what you are doing. Try not to show anxiety; act with confidence. Your calm behavior can help reassure the sick person.

If there are two or more rescuers, one should obtain emergency assistance while the other is following the procedures outlined below.

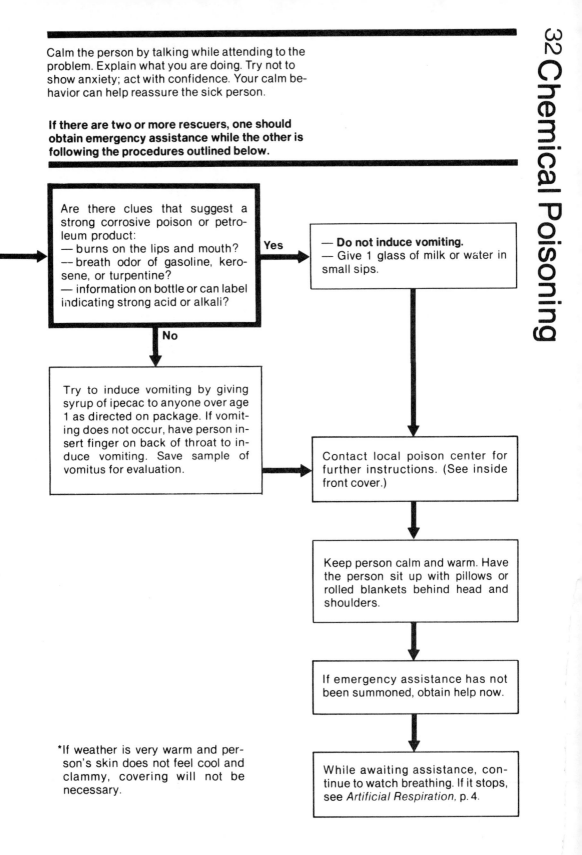

Are there clues that suggest a strong corrosive poison or petroleum product:
— burns on the lips and mouth?
— breath odor of gasoline, kerosene, or turpentine?
— information on bottle or can label indicating strong acid or alkali?

Yes

— **Do not induce vomiting.**
— Give 1 glass of milk or water in small sips.

No

Try to induce vomiting by giving syrup of ipecac to anyone over age 1 as directed on package. If vomiting does not occur, have person insert finger on back of throat to induce vomiting. Save sample of vomitus for evaluation.

Contact local poison center for further instructions. (See inside front cover.)

Keep person calm and warm. Have the person sit up with pillows or rolled blankets behind head and shoulders.

If emergency assistance has not been summoned, obtain help now.

*If weather is very warm and person's skin does not feel cool and clammy, covering will not be necessary.

While awaiting assistance, continue to watch breathing. If it stops, see *Artificial Respiration*, p. 4.

33 Chest Injury

For *Chest Pain* without injury, see p. 13.

If there was a severe blow to the head or a fall, or if person is unconscious, assume neck injury and do not move.

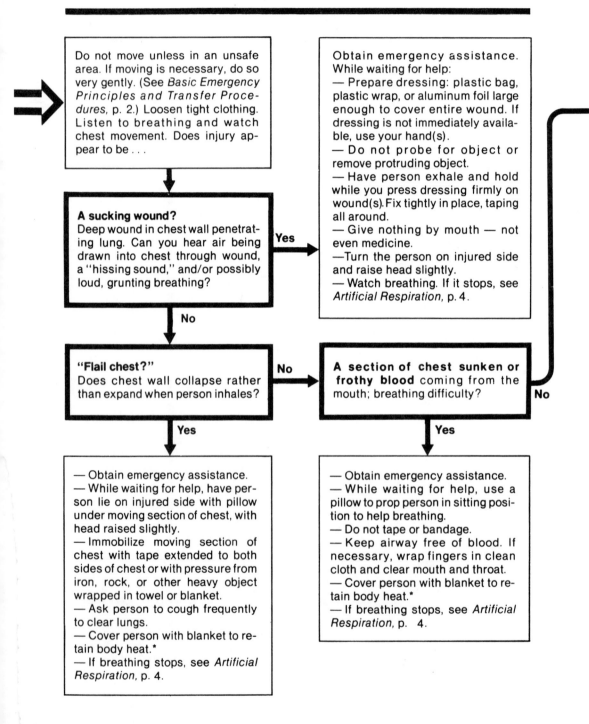

Do not move unless in an unsafe area. If moving is necessary, do so very gently. (See *Basic Emergency Principles and Transfer Procedures,* p. 2.) Loosen tight clothing. Listen to breathing and watch chest movement. Does injury appear to be . . .

A sucking wound?
Deep wound in chest wall penetrating lung. Can you hear air being drawn into chest through wound, a "hissing sound," and/or possibly loud, grunting breathing?

→ **Yes**

Obtain emergency assistance. While waiting for help:
— Prepare dressing: plastic bag, plastic wrap, or aluminum foil large enough to cover entire wound. If dressing is not immediately available, use your hand(s).
— Do not probe for object or remove protruding object.
— Have person exhale and hold while you press dressing firmly on wound(s). Fix tightly in place, taping all around.
— Give nothing by mouth — not even medicine.
—Turn the person on injured side and raise head slightly.
— Watch breathing. If it stops, see *Artificial Respiration,* p. 4.

No

"Flail chest?"
Does chest wall collapse rather than expand when person inhales?

→ **No** →

A section of chest sunken or frothy blood coming from the mouth; breathing difficulty?

No

Yes

— Obtain emergency assistance.
— While waiting for help, have person lie on injured side with pillow under moving section of chest, with head raised slightly.
— Immobilize moving section of chest with tape extended to both sides of chest or with pressure from iron, rock, or other heavy object wrapped in towel or blanket.
— Ask person to cough frequently to clear lungs.
— Cover person with blanket to retain body heat.*
— If breathing stops, see *Artificial Respiration,* p. 4.

Yes

— Obtain emergency assistance.
— While waiting for help, use a pillow to prop person in sitting position to help breathing.
— Do not tape or bandage.
— Keep airway free of blood. If necessary, wrap fingers in clean cloth and clear mouth and throat.
— Cover person with blanket to retain body heat.*
— If breathing stops, see *Artificial Respiration,* p. 4.

Calm the person by talking while attending to the problem. Explain what you are doing. Try not to show anxiety; act with confidence. Your calm behavior can help to reassure the injured person.

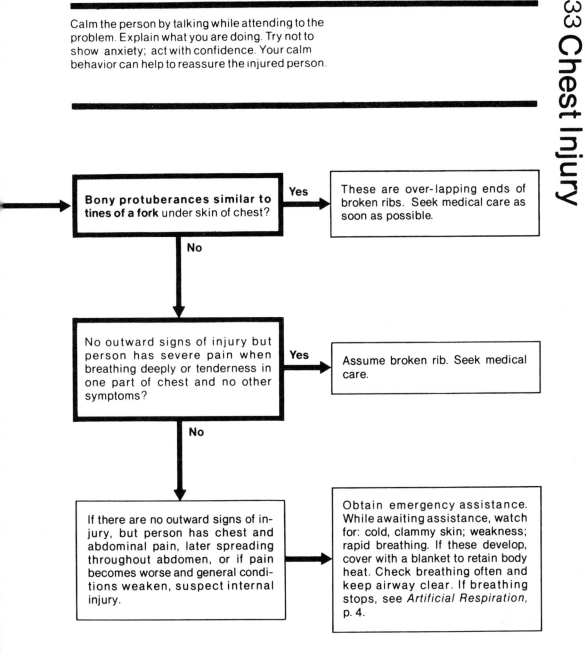

Bony protuberances similar to tines of a fork under skin of chest?

Yes → These are over-lapping ends of broken ribs. Seek medical care as soon as possible.

No

No outward signs of injury but person has severe pain when breathing deeply or tenderness in one part of chest and no other symptoms?

Yes → Assume broken rib. Seek medical care.

No

If there are no outward signs of injury, but person has chest and abdominal pain, later spreading throughout abdomen, or if pain becomes worse and general conditions weaken, suspect internal injury.

→ Obtain emergency assistance. While awaiting assistance, watch for: cold, clammy skin; weakness; rapid breathing. If these develop, cover with a blanket to retain body heat. Check breathing often and keep airway clear. If breathing stops, see *Artificial Respiration,* p. 4.

*If weather is very warm and person's skin does not feel cool and clammy, covering will not be necessary.

Minor Cuts
(Including Rope Burns)

Definition: *minor bleeding/no involvement of underlying tissue (nerve, muscle, tendon, artery, vein)*

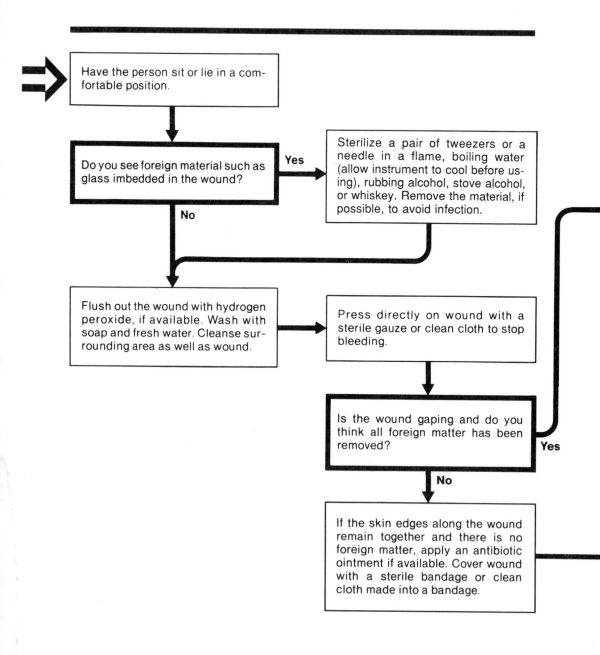

Have the person sit or lie in a comfortable position.

Do you see foreign material such as glass imbedded in the wound?

Yes → Sterilize a pair of tweezers or a needle in a flame, boiling water (allow instrument to cool before using), rubbing alcohol, stove alcohol, or whiskey. Remove the material, if possible, to avoid infection.

No

Flush out the wound with hydrogen peroxide, if available. Wash with soap and fresh water. Cleanse surrounding area as well as wound.

→ Press directly on wound with a sterile gauze or clean cloth to stop bleeding.

Is the wound gaping and do you think all foreign matter has been removed?

Yes

No

If the skin edges along the wound remain together and there is no foreign matter, apply an antibiotic ointment if available. Cover wound with a sterile bandage or clean cloth made into a bandage.

Calm the person by talking while attending to the problem. Explain what you are doing. Try not to show anxiety; act with confidence. Your calm behavior can help to reassure the injured person.

If injury was the result of a vehicular or job-related accident, the person should be examined by a physician for possible additional injuries or complications.

Form a butterfly strip from adhesive tape. Draw the skin edges together and use the strips to close the wound. No other dressing should be necessary unless wound is on foot, then pad with gauze and tape in place.

Seek medical care as soon as possible. Person may require sutures and/or tetanus immunization.

Butterfly strip

Take a strip of adhesive tape about 3½ inches long . . . Make four cuts (slightly inward) and fold in, sticky side to sticky side.

If person has not received tetanus shot within 3-5 years, if wound is very dirty or has foreign matter, or if any signs of infection develop (redness, swelling, etc.), seek medical care.

35 Dislocations

Signs & Symptoms: *distortion in shape of joint/ swelling and discoloration/pain with movement/ affected limb looks longer or shorter/loss of movement in joint.*
If you suspect Back or Neck Injury, see p. 29.

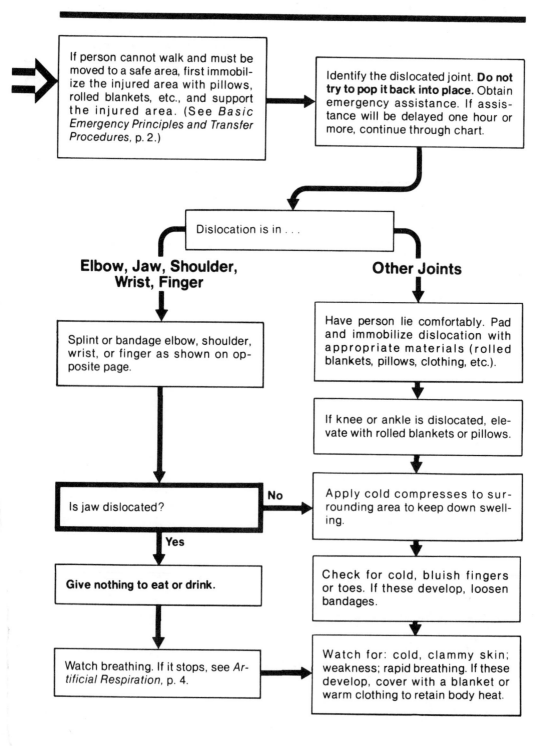

If person cannot walk and must be moved to a safe area, first immobilize the injured area with pillows, rolled blankets, etc., and support the injured area. (See *Basic Emergency Principles and Transfer Procedures*, p. 2.)

Identify the dislocated joint. **Do not try to pop it back into place.** Obtain emergency assistance. If assistance will be delayed one hour or more, continue through chart.

Dislocation is in . . .

Elbow, Jaw, Shoulder, Wrist, Finger

Other Joints

Splint or bandage elbow, shoulder, wrist, or finger as shown on opposite page.

Have person lie comfortably. Pad and immobilize dislocation with appropriate materials (rolled blankets, pillows, clothing, etc.).

If knee or ankle is dislocated, elevate with rolled blankets or pillows.

Is jaw dislocated? **No** → Apply cold compresses to surrounding area to keep down swelling.

Yes

Give nothing to eat or drink.

Check for cold, bluish fingers or toes. If these develop, loosen bandages.

Watch breathing. If it stops, see *Artificial Respiration*, p. 4.

Watch for: cold, clammy skin; weakness; rapid breathing. If these develop, cover with a blanket or warm clothing to retain body heat.

Calm the person by talking while attending to the problem. Explain what you are doing. Try not to show anxiety; act with confidence. Your calm behavior can help to reassure the injured person.

Finger

splints: eating spoons, padded stick, other finger.

Elbow, Shoulder, or Wrist Sling

suggested materials:
shirt or jacket
large handkerchief, towel, bandana, or piece of sheet folded diagonally.

Tie together behind neck.

Pin flap up.

If shoulder is dislocated, bandage upper arm against chest wall over sling

36 Chemical Burns of the Eyes

**If there are two or more rescuers, one should
obtain emergency assistance while the other is
following the procedures outlined below.**

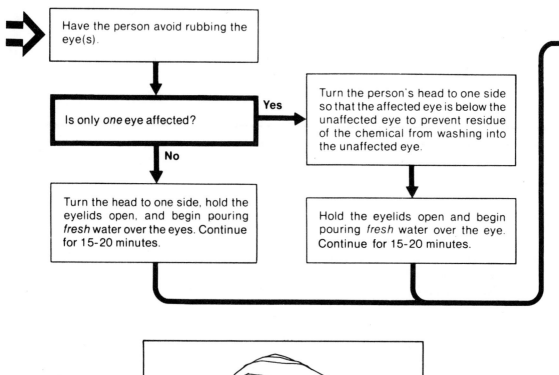

Have the person avoid rubbing the eye(s).

Is only *one* eye affected?

Yes → Turn the person's head to one side so that the affected eye is below the unaffected eye to prevent residue of the chemical from washing into the unaffected eye.

No

Turn the head to one side, hold the eyelids open, and begin pouring *fresh* water over the eyes. Continue for 15-20 minutes.

Hold the eyelids open and begin pouring *fresh* water over the eye. Continue for 15-20 minutes.

Calm the person by talking while attending to the problem. Explain what you are doing. Try not to show anxiety; act with confidence. Your calm behavior can help to reassure the injured person.

Remove the coagulated chemical from the eye with moistened sterile gauze.

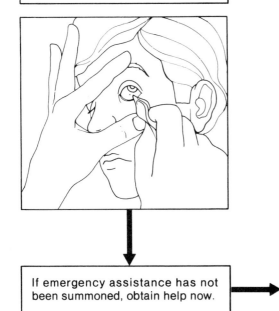

If emergency assistance has not been summoned, obtain help now.

While awaiting assistance, continue to rinse out the eye(s) until help arrives.

37 Foreign Object in Eye
(With no injury or bleeding)

For chemicals in eye, see *Chemical Burns of the Eyes*, **p. 36.**

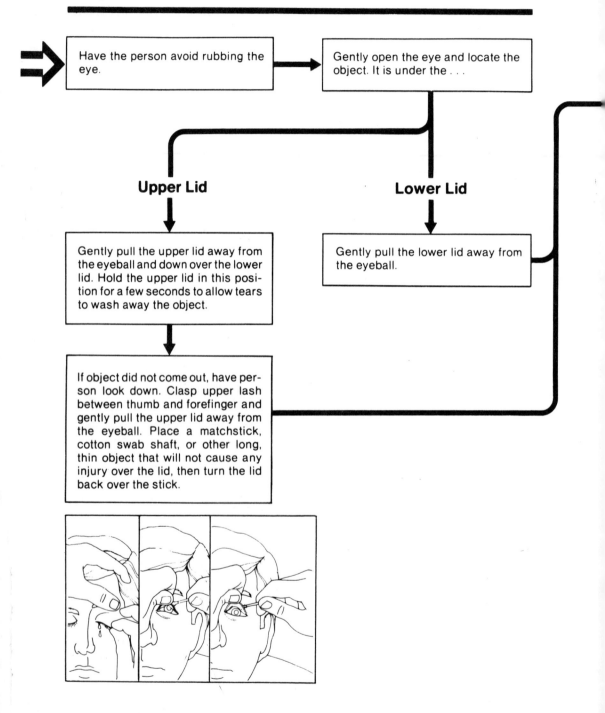

Have the person avoid rubbing the eye.

Gently open the eye and locate the object. It is under the . . .

Upper Lid

Lower Lid

Gently pull the upper lid away from the eyeball and down over the lower lid. Hold the upper lid in this position for a few seconds to allow tears to wash away the object.

Gently pull the lower lid away from the eyeball.

If object did not come out, have person look down. Clasp upper lash between thumb and forefinger and gently pull the upper lid away from the eyeball. Place a matchstick, cotton swab shaft, or other long, thin object that will not cause any injury over the lid, then turn the lid back over the stick.

Calm the person by talking while attending to the problem. Explain what you are doing. Try not to show anxiety; act with confidence. Your calm behavior can help to reassure the injured person.

Is the foreign object on the *inside* of the lid?

Yes

Gently remove it with a moistened tissue or cloth or by pouring fresh water in eye. No further treatment will be necessary unless swelling, pain, or discoloration develop. If these occur, seek medical care.

No

If you think the object is imbedded in the cornea, do not attempt to remove it. Cover both eyes with a dry bandage. **Do not apply any pressure.** Seek medical care.

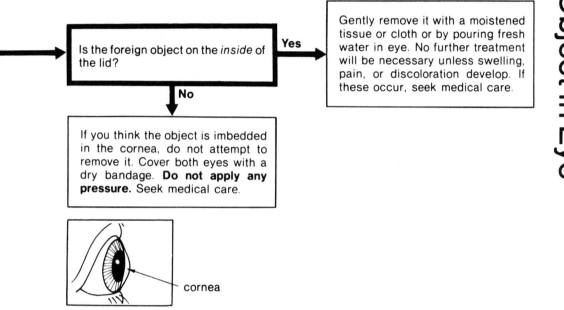

cornea

38 Eye Injury

For chemicals in the eye, see p. 36. For small foreign object in eye, but not penetrating eye, see p. 37.

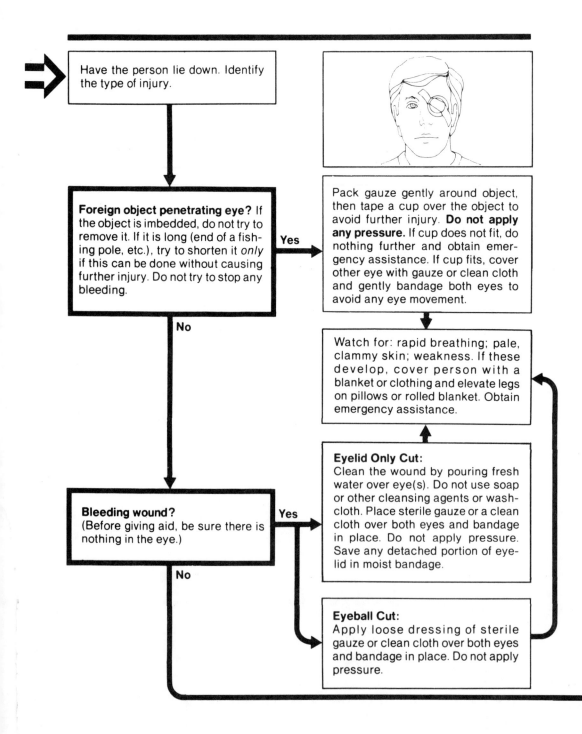

Have the person lie down. Identify the type of injury.

Foreign object penetrating eye? If the object is imbedded, do not try to remove it. If it is long (end of a fishing pole, etc.), try to shorten it *only* if this can be done without causing further injury. Do not try to stop any bleeding.

Yes → Pack gauze gently around object, then tape a cup over the object to avoid further injury. **Do not apply any pressure.** If cup does not fit, do nothing further and obtain emergency assistance. If cup fits, cover other eye with gauze or clean cloth and gently bandage both eyes to avoid any eye movement.

No

Watch for: rapid breathing; pale, clammy skin; weakness. If these develop, cover person with a blanket or clothing and elevate legs on pillows or rolled blanket. Obtain emergency assistance.

Bleeding wound?
(Before giving aid, be sure there is nothing in the eye.)

Yes → **Eyelid Only Cut:**
Clean the wound by pouring fresh water over eye(s). Do not use soap or other cleansing agents or washcloth. Place sterile gauze or a clean cloth over both eyes and bandage in place. Do not apply pressure. Save any detached portion of eyelid in moist bandage.

No

Eyeball Cut:
Apply loose dressing of sterile gauze or clean cloth over both eyes and bandage in place. Do not apply pressure.

Calm the person by talking while attending to the problem. Explain what you are doing. Try not to show anxiety; act with confidence. Your calm behavior can help to reassure the injured person. **If injury was the result of a vehicular or job-related accident, the person should be examined by a physician for possible additional injuries or complications.**

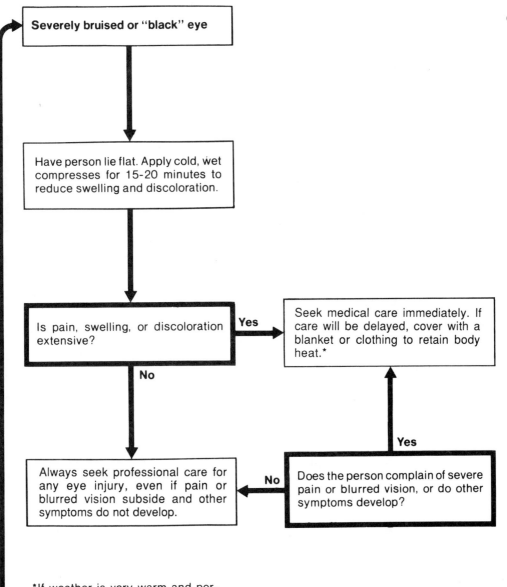

Severely bruised or "black" eye

Have person lie flat. Apply cold, wet compresses for 15-20 minutes to reduce swelling and discoloration.

Is pain, swelling, or discoloration extensive?

Yes → Seek medical care immediately. If care will be delayed, cover with a blanket or clothing to retain body heat.*

No ↓

Always seek professional care for any eye injury, even if pain or blurred vision subside and other symptoms do not develop.

No ← Does the person complain of severe pain or blurred vision, or do other symptoms develop?

Yes ↑

*If weather is very warm and person's skin does not feel cool and clammy, covering will not be necessary.

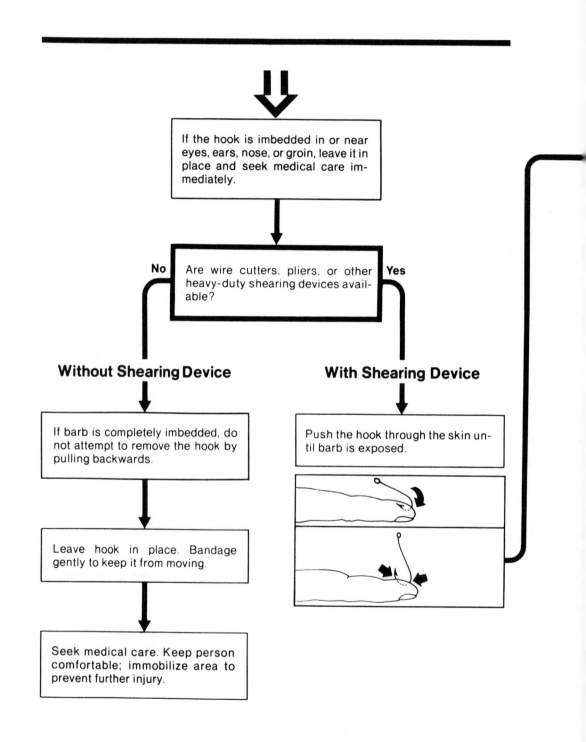

If the hook is imbedded in or near eyes, ears, nose, or groin, leave it in place and seek medical care immediately.

No   Are wire cutters, pliers, or other heavy-duty shearing devices available?   **Yes**

Without Shearing Device

If barb is completely imbedded, do not attempt to remove the hook by pulling backwards.

Leave hook in place. Bandage gently to keep it from moving.

Seek medical care. Keep person comfortable; immobilize area to prevent further injury.

With Shearing Device

Push the hook through the skin until barb is exposed.

Calm the person by talking while attending to the problem. Explain what you are doing. Try not to show anxiety; act with confidence. Your calm behavior can help to reassure the injured person.

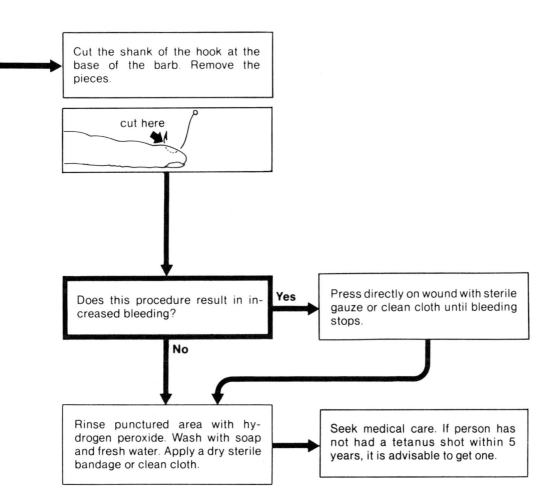

Cut the shank of the hook at the base of the barb. Remove the pieces.

cut here

Does this procedure result in increased bleeding?

Yes → Press directly on wound with sterile gauze or clean cloth until bleeding stops.

No

Rinse punctured area with hydrogen peroxide. Wash with soap and fresh water. Apply a dry sterile bandage or clean cloth.

→ Seek medical care. If person has not had a tetanus shot within 5 years, it is advisable to get one.

40 Food Poisoning

If there are two or more rescuers, one should obtain emergency assistance while the other is following the procedures outlined below.

Signs & Symptoms: *nausea/possible vomiting/ chills/diarrhea/cramps/recent ingestion of food that "didn't taste right" or was old or otherwise suspect/others with same symptoms. See other symptoms in chart.*
For food allergy, see *Allergic Reaction*, **p. 27.**

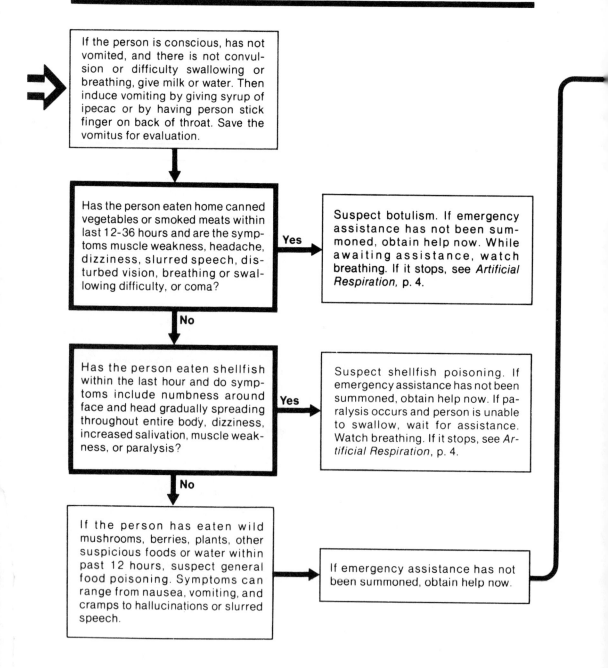

If the person is conscious, has not vomited, and there is not convulsion or difficulty swallowing or breathing, give milk or water. Then induce vomiting by giving syrup of ipecac or by having person stick finger on back of throat. Save the vomitus for evaluation.

Has the person eaten home canned vegetables or smoked meats within last 12-36 hours and are the symptoms muscle weakness, headache, dizziness, slurred speech, disturbed vision, breathing or swallowing difficulty, or coma?

Yes → Suspect botulism. If emergency assistance has not been summoned, obtain help now. While awaiting assistance, watch breathing. If it stops, see *Artificial Respiration*, p. 4.

No

Has the person eaten shellfish within the last hour and do symptoms include numbness around face and head gradually spreading throughout entire body, dizziness, increased salivation, muscle weakness, or paralysis?

Yes → Suspect shellfish poisoning. If emergency assistance has not been summoned, obtain help now. If paralysis occurs and person is unable to swallow, wait for assistance. Watch breathing. If it stops, see *Artificial Respiration*, p. 4.

No

If the person has eaten wild mushrooms, berries, plants, other suspicious foods or water within past 12 hours, suspect general food poisoning. Symptoms can range from nausea, vomiting, and cramps to hallucinations or slurred speech.

→ If emergency assistance has not been summoned, obtain help now.

Calm the person by talking while attending to the problem. Explain what you are doing. Try not to show anxiety; act with confidence. Your calm behavior can help to reassure the sick person.

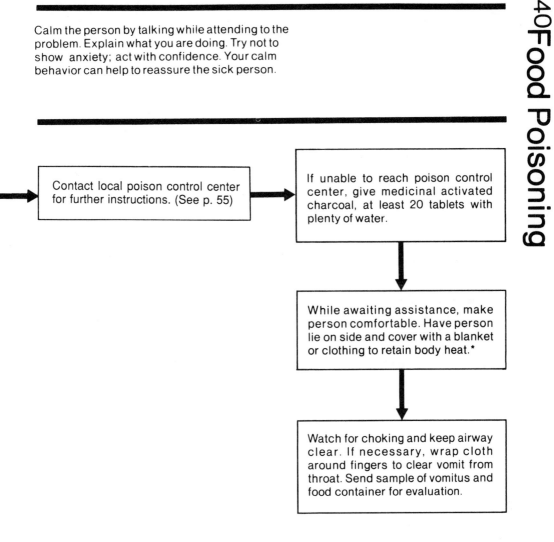

Contact local poison control center for further instructions. (See p. 55)

If unable to reach poison control center, give medicinal activated charcoal, at least 20 tablets with plenty of water.

While awaiting assistance, make person comfortable. Have person lie on side and cover with a blanket or clothing to retain body heat.*

Watch for choking and keep airway clear. If necessary, wrap cloth around fingers to clear vomit from throat. Send sample of vomitus and food container for evaluation.

*If weather is very warm and person's skin does not feel cool and clammy, covering will not be necessary.

41 Fractures

For *Severe Head Injury*, see p. 42.
For *Back or Neck Injuries*, see p. 29

Signs & Symptoms: *sound of bone snapping/ deformity with swelling and discoloration/ painful to touch/possible grating sensation of broken bone ends. With any injury, if you're not sure, assume there is a fracture.*

If there are two or more rescuers, one should obtain emergency assistance while the other is following the procedures outlined below.

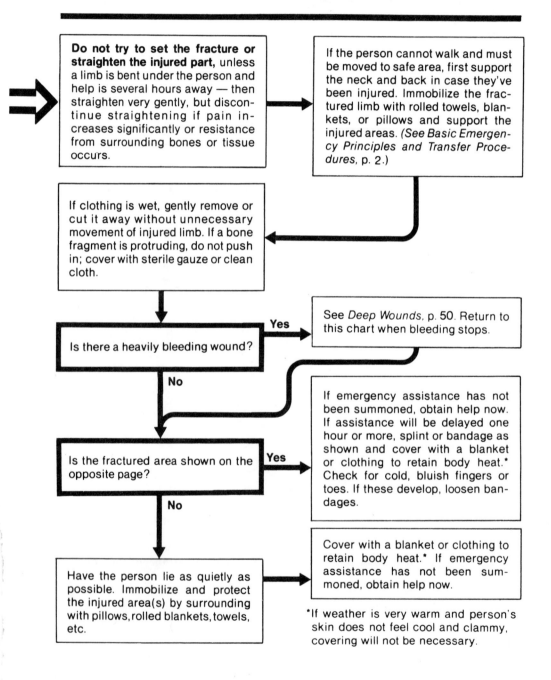

Do not try to set the fracture or straighten the injured part, unless a limb is bent under the person and help is several hours away — then straighten very gently, but discontinue straightening if pain increases significantly or resistance from surrounding bones or tissue occurs.

If the person cannot walk and must be moved to safe area, first support the neck and back in case they've been injured. Immobilize the fractured limb with rolled towels, blankets, or pillows and support the injured areas. *(See Basic Emergency Principles and Transfer Procedures, p. 2.)*

If clothing is wet, gently remove or cut it away without unnecessary movement of injured limb. If a bone fragment is protruding, do not push in; cover with sterile gauze or clean cloth.

Is there a heavily bleeding wound?

Yes → See *Deep Wounds*, p. 50. Return to this chart when bleeding stops.

No

Is the fractured area shown on the opposite page?

Yes → If emergency assistance has not been summoned, obtain help now. If assistance will be delayed one hour or more, splint or bandage as shown and cover with a blanket or clothing to retain body heat.* Check for cold, bluish fingers or toes. If these develop, loosen bandages.

No

Have the person lie as quietly as possible. Immobilize and protect the injured area(s) by surrounding with pillows, rolled blankets, towels, etc.

Cover with a blanket or clothing to retain body heat.* If emergency assistance has not been summoned, obtain help now.

*If weather is very warm and person's skin does not feel cool and clammy, covering will not be necessary.

Calm the person by talking while attending to the problem. Explain what you are doing. Try not to show anxiety; act with confidence. Your calm behavior can help to reassure the injured person.

Upper Arm

splints: rolled magazines, newspapers, or heavy cardboard; cooking spoons, garden stakes, or tool handles wrapped in sheeting, towels, or shirts for padding. sling: sheeting, large handkerchief, or towel folded diagonally.

Lash one or two splints to upper arm from elbow to shoulder.

Lay forearm across chest and hold in a sling.

Secure upper arm to chest with two bandages.

Forearm, wrist, or hand

Use rolled handkerchief as pad to be grasped in hand, then splint as for upper arm and put in sling.

Elbow splint

Suggested materials for splint: Same as for upper arm.

Collarbone

Make sling and secure as shown.

Ankle and Foot

Pad injured part firmly with blanket, towels, or pillow. Secure with tape or strips of cloth. Keep leg elevated.

Finger

splints: eating spoon, padded stick, other finger.

42 Severe Head Injury

Signs & Symptoms
Skull Fracture: *dizziness/double vision/ slurred speech/headache/possible bleeding or draining of clear fluid from ears, nose, or mouth/possible nausea and vomiting/possible convulsions/ pupils of unequal size/paralysis on the side opposite injury/deformity of skull/unconscious- ness. One eye may appear sunken.*

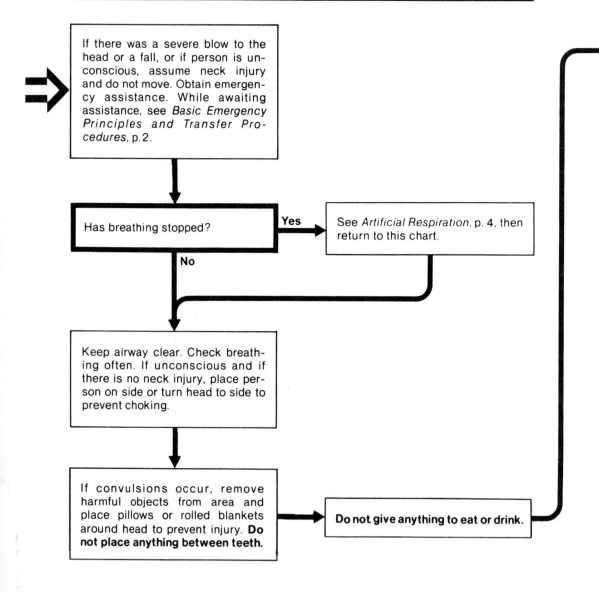

If there was a severe blow to the head or a fall, or if person is unconscious, assume neck injury and do not move. Obtain emergency assistance. While awaiting assistance, see *Basic Emergency Principles and Transfer Procedures*, p. 2.

Has breathing stopped? — **Yes** → See *Artificial Respiration*, p. 4, then return to this chart.

No

Keep airway clear. Check breathing often. If unconscious and if there is no neck injury, place person on side or turn head to side to prevent choking.

If convulsions occur, remove harmful objects from area and place pillows or rolled blankets around head to prevent injury. **Do not place anything between teeth.**

Do not give anything to eat or drink.

Calm the person by talking while attending to the problem. Explain what you are doing. Try not to show anxiety; act with confidence. Your calm behavior can help to reassure the injured person.

If there are two or more rescuers, one should obtain emergency assistance while the other is following the procedures outlined below.

Is there an open wound?

Yes → Cover wound with a thick, sterile gauze pad or clean cloth. Use a strip of cloth or bandage to hold pad in place. Take another strip and wrap it around head and over pad while pulling gently but firmly. Do not press directly on wound and do not move head if neck injury is suspected.

See illustration below.

No ↓

Keep person quiet. Cover with a blanket to retain body heat.* If there is no neck injury, have person lie with a rolled blanket or pillow beneath head and shoulders. Keep mouth clear of blood and vomit.

↓

Obtain emergency assistance if not already summoned.

→ While awaiting assistance, continue to watch breathing. If it stops, see *Artificial Respiration,* p.4.

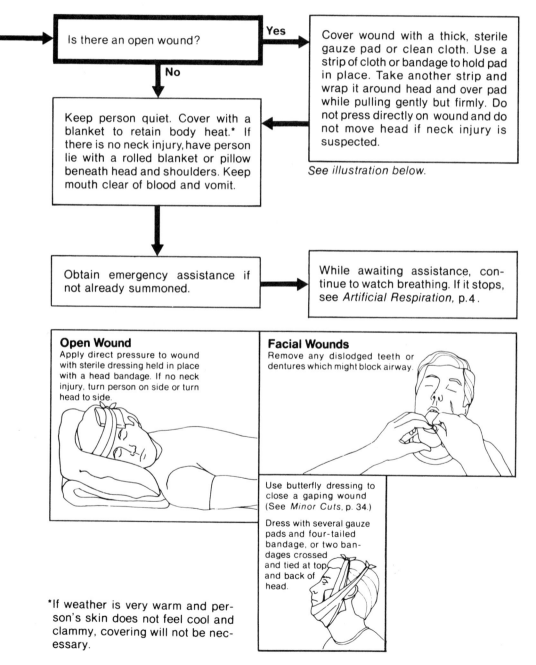

Open Wound
Apply direct pressure to wound with sterile dressing held in place with a head bandage. If no neck injury, turn person on side or turn head to side.

Facial Wounds
Remove any dislodged teeth or dentures which might block airway.

Use butterfly dressing to close a gaping wound (See *Minor Cuts,* p. 34.)

Dress with several gauze pads and four-tailed bandage, or two bandages crossed and tied at top and back of head.

*If weather is very warm and person's skin does not feel cool and clammy, covering will not be necessary.

43 Inhaled Poisons

(Including Carbon Monoxide, Carbon Dioxide, Ammonia, Chlorine, Natural Gas, Anesthetics, and other gases and fumes)

Signs & Symptoms: *different breath odor/dizziness/headache/irritability/ difficulty breathing/nausea/vomiting/ diarrhea/faintness/pale, bluish or bright red lips and skin/unconsciousness*

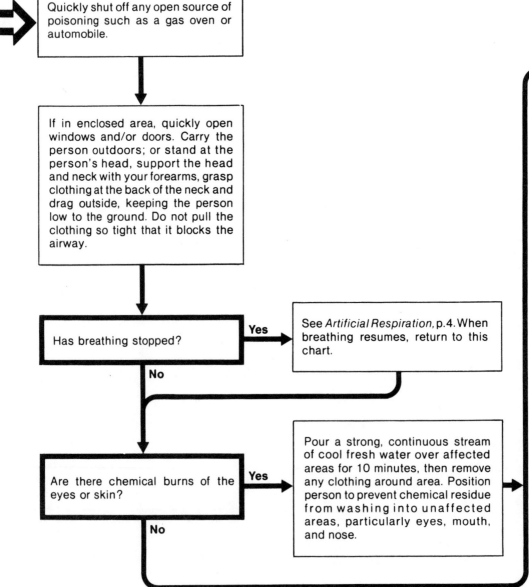

Quickly shut off any open source of poisoning such as a gas oven or automobile.

If in enclosed area, quickly open windows and/or doors. Carry the person outdoors; or stand at the person's head, support the head and neck with your forearms, grasp clothing at the back of the neck and drag outside, keeping the person low to the ground. Do not pull the clothing so tight that it blocks the airway.

Has breathing stopped? — **Yes** → See *Artificial Respiration*, p. 4. When breathing resumes, return to this chart.

No

Are there chemical burns of the eyes or skin? — **Yes** → Pour a strong, continuous stream of cool fresh water over affected areas for 10 minutes, then remove any clothing around area. Position person to prevent chemical residue from washing into unaffected areas, particularly eyes, mouth, and nose.

No

Calm the person by talking while attending to the problem. Explain what you are doing. Try not to show anxiety; act with confidence. Your calm behavior can help to reassure the injured person.

If there are two or more rescuers, one should obtain emergency assistance and request oxygen while the other is following the procedures outlined below.

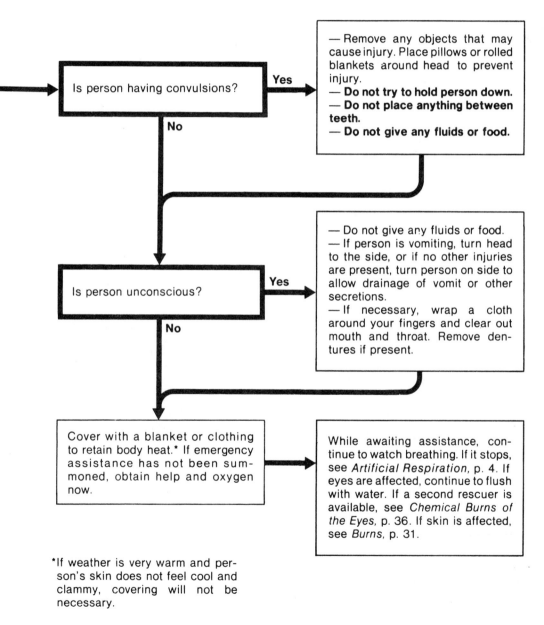

Is person having convulsions?

Yes

— Remove any objects that may cause injury. Place pillows or rolled blankets around head to prevent injury.
— **Do not try to hold person down.**
— **Do not place anything between teeth.**
— **Do not give any fluids or food.**

No

Is person unconscious?

Yes

— Do not give any fluids or food.
— If person is vomiting, turn head to the side, or if no other injuries are present, turn person on side to allow drainage of vomit or other secretions.
— If necessary, wrap a cloth around your fingers and clear out mouth and throat. Remove dentures if present.

No

Cover with a blanket or clothing to retain body heat.* If emergency assistance has not been summoned, obtain help and oxygen now.

While awaiting assistance, continue to watch breathing. If it stops, see *Artificial Respiration*, p. 4. If eyes are affected, continue to flush with water. If a second rescuer is available, see *Chemical Burns of the Eyes*, p. 36. If skin is affected, see *Burns*, p. 31.

*If weather is very warm and person's skin does not feel cool and clammy, covering will not be necessary.

44 Insect Stings

Signs & Symptoms
Emergency allergic reaction: breathing difficulty/
faintness/cool or moist skin/swollen, red, teary
eyes/hives/blotches/swollen nasal passages/
nausea/vomiting/diarrhea (Very serious reactions
with wheezing and collapse are apt to occur within 5-10 minutes.)
Less serious: local irritation or pain/moderate
swelling/local redness or itching

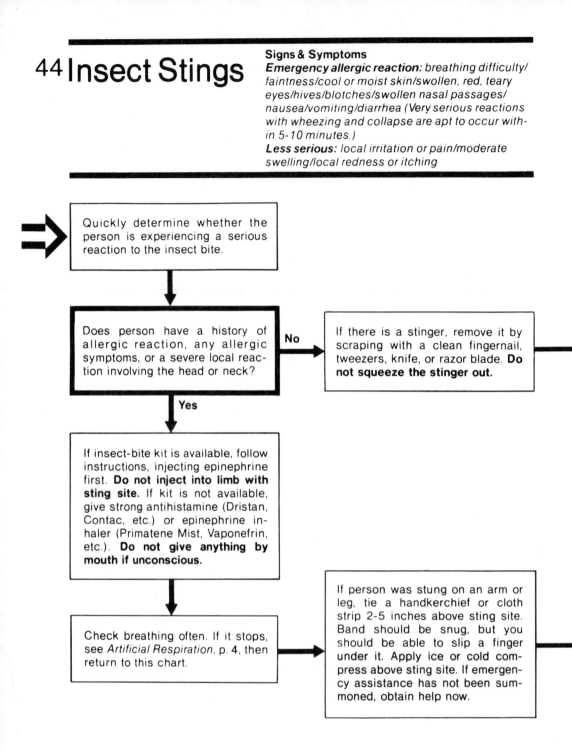

Quickly determine whether the person is experiencing a serious reaction to the insect bite.

Does person have a history of allergic reaction, any allergic symptoms, or a severe local reaction involving the head or neck?

No → If there is a stinger, remove it by scraping with a clean fingernail, tweezers, knife, or razor blade. **Do not squeeze the stinger out.**

Yes

If insect-bite kit is available, follow instructions, injecting epinephrine first. **Do not inject into limb with sting site.** If kit is not available, give strong antihistamine (Dristan, Contac, etc.) or epinephrine inhaler (Primatene Mist, Vaponefrin, etc.). **Do not give anything by mouth if unconscious.**

Check breathing often. If it stops, see *Artificial Respiration*, p. 4, then return to this chart.

If person was stung on an arm or leg, tie a handkerchief or cloth strip 2-5 inches above sting site. Band should be snug, but you should be able to slip a finger under it. Apply ice or cold compress above sting site. If emergency assistance has not been summoned, obtain help now.

Calm the person by talking while attending to the problem. Explain what you are doing. Try not to show anxiety; act with confidence. Your calm behavior can help to reassure the injured person.

For emergency allergic reaction, when there are two or more rescuers, one should obtain emergency assistance while the other is following the procedures outlined below.

Wash sting site with soap and water. Apply cold compresses for 15-20 minutes, then apply calamine lotion or meat tenderizer mixed with water to make a thick paste.

Watch for signs of infection or any allergic symptoms that may develop. If they appear, seek medical care.

Keep person quiet and calm. Loosen the band for a few seconds every 3-5 minutes. Remove after 30 minutes. Keep bite site below heart level.

While awaiting assistance, continue to watch breathing. If it stops, see *Artificial Respiration*, p. 4.

45 Poison Ivy, Oak, & Sumac

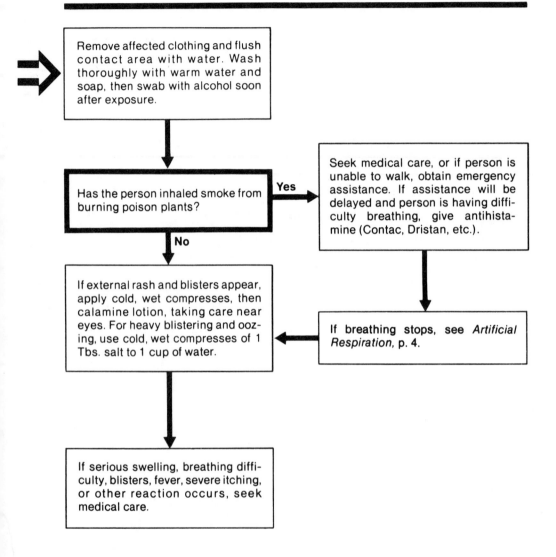

Remove affected clothing and flush contact area with water. Wash thoroughly with warm water and soap, then swab with alcohol soon after exposure.

Has the person inhaled smoke from burning poison plants?

Yes

Seek medical care, or if person is unable to walk, obtain emergency assistance. If assistance will be delayed and person is having difficulty breathing, give antihistamine (Contac, Dristan, etc.).

No

If external rash and blisters appear, apply cold, wet compresses, then calamine lotion, taking care near eyes. For heavy blistering and oozing, use cold, wet compresses of 1 Tbs. salt to 1 cup of water.

If breathing stops, see *Artificial Respiration*, p. 4.

If serious swelling, breathing difficulty, blisters, fever, severe itching, or other reaction occurs, seek medical care.

Calm the person by talking while attending to the problem. Explain what you are doing. Try not to show concern; act with confidence. Your calm behavior can help to reassure the injured person.

Recognize common poison plants:

Poison Ivy
Small plant, vine, or shrub common throughout U.S. except California. Shiny leaves grow in clusters of three, turning red and yellow toward Fall.

Poison Oak
Western variety grows in California and portions of adjacent states as shrub or vine closely resembling poison ivy.
More common variety grows in other areas, usually as a shrub with clusters of hairy, yellowish berries and undersides of leaves covered with hair.

Poison Sumac
Woody shrub or small tree (5-25 feet) grows in eastern U.S., especially in moist climates.
Each leaf stalk has 7-13 leaflets with smooth edges, which turn red in Fall, and cream-colored berries which hang from branches in loose clusters.

46 Snakebite

These procedures must be followed *immediately* after snakebite.

Signs & Symptoms:
Poisonous: *Severe reaction occurs within 30 minutes. Burning pain at bite/swelling/discoloration/ weakness/dizziness/faint pulse. Coral snake reactions may appear less severe and may be delayed up to 18 hours. See maps and descriptions of poisonous snakes, next page.*

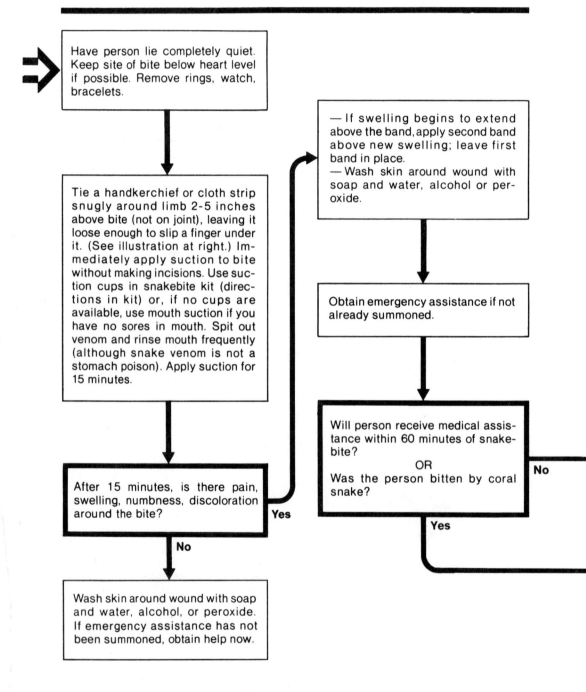

Have person lie completely quiet. Keep site of bite below heart level if possible. Remove rings, watch, bracelets.

Tie a handkerchief or cloth strip snugly around limb 2-5 inches above bite (not on joint), leaving it loose enough to slip a finger under it. (See illustration at right.) Immediately apply suction to bite without making incisions. Use suction cups in snakebite kit (directions in kit) or, if no cups are available, use mouth suction if you have no sores in mouth. Spit out venom and rinse mouth frequently (although snake venom is not a stomach poison). Apply suction for 15 minutes.

After 15 minutes, is there pain, swelling, numbness, discoloration around the bite?

No

Yes

Wash skin around wound with soap and water, alcohol, or peroxide. If emergency assistance has not been summoned, obtain help now.

— If swelling begins to extend above the band, apply second band above new swelling; leave first band in place.
— Wash skin around wound with soap and water, alcohol or peroxide.

Obtain emergency assistance if not already summoned.

Will person receive medical assistance within 60 minutes of snakebite?
OR
Was the person bitten by coral snake?

No

Yes

Calm the person by talking while attending to the problem. Explain what you are doing. Try not to show anxiety; act with confidence. Your calm behavior can help to reassure the injured person.

If there are two or more rescuers, one should obtain emergency assistance while the other is following the procedures outlined below.

—Sterilize knife or razor blade with alcohol or by holding in a flame.
—Make a linear, *not crosswise,* incision through each fang mark, about ⅛ to ¼ inch long, not more than ⅛ inch deep. **Do not** cut deeply enough to damage nerves or muscles. **Do not** cut through a vein. *(See illustration below.)*

— Apply suction with cups in snakebite kit. (Directions in kit.) If not enough cups to cover all incisions, rotate them every 3-5 minutes. If no cups are available, use mouth suction if you have no open sores in mouth. Spit out venom and rinse mouth frequently (although snake venom is not a stomach poison).

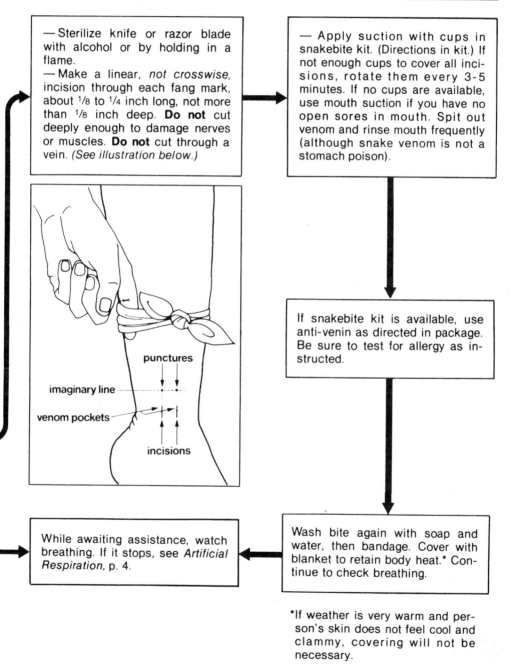

If snakebite kit is available, use anti-venin as directed in package. Be sure to test for allergy as instructed.

While awaiting assistance, watch breathing. If it stops, see *Artificial Respiration,* p. 4.

Wash bite again with soap and water, then bandage. Cover with blanket to retain body heat.* Continue to check breathing.

*If weather is very warm and person's skin does not feel cool and clammy, covering will not be necessary.

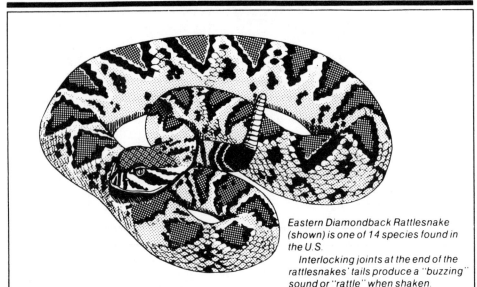

Eastern Diamondback Rattlesnake (shown) is one of 14 species found in the U.S.

Interlocking joints at the end of the rattlesnakes' tails produce a "buzzing" sound or "rattle" when shaken.

Eastern Diamondback Rattlesnake

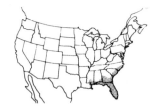

Description Dark diamonds with light borders along a tan or light brown background. Diamonds gradually changing to bands in tail. Diagonal brown lines on the sides of face, vertical on snout.
Habitat Lowland thickets, palmettos, flatwoods.

Canebrake and Timber Rattlesnake

Description South: Dark streak from canebrake snake's eye to mouth; dark chevrons and rusty stripe along midline. Pink to tan ground color darker toward tail, which is black in adults. North: timber rattlesnake has yellowish ground color and a dark phase in part of its range.
Habitat Canebrake: lowland brush, and stream borders. Timber rattlesnake: rocky wooded hills.

Western Diamondback Rattlesnake

Description Light brown to black diamond-shaped blotches along light grey, tan, and, in some localities, pink background. Black and white bands of about equal width around tail and black basal rattle.
Habitat Diverse terrain: dry, sparsely wooded, rocky hills, flat desert and coastal sand dunes. Often found in agricultural land and near towns.

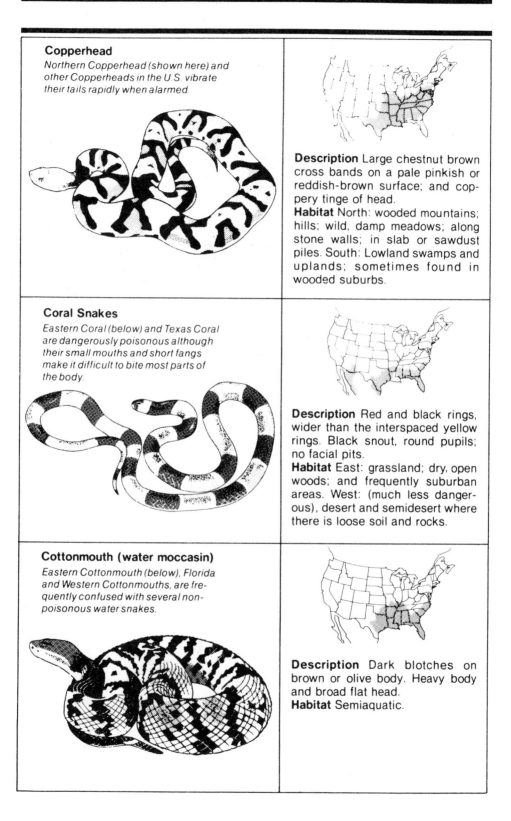

Copperhead

Northern Copperhead (shown here) and other Copperheads in the U.S. vibrate their tails rapidly when alarmed.

Description Large chestnut brown cross bands on a pale pinkish or reddish-brown surface; and coppery tinge of head.
Habitat North: wooded mountains; hills; wild, damp meadows; along stone walls; in slab or sawdust piles. South: Lowland swamps and uplands; sometimes found in wooded suburbs.

Coral Snakes

Eastern Coral (below) and Texas Coral are dangerously poisonous although their small mouths and short fangs make it difficult to bite most parts of the body.

Description Red and black rings, wider than the interspaced yellow rings. Black snout, round pupils; no facial pits.
Habitat East: grassland; dry, open woods; and frequently suburban areas. West: (much less dangerous), desert and semidesert where there is loose soil and rocks.

Cottonmouth (water moccasin)

Eastern Cottonmouth (below), Florida and Western Cottonmouths, are frequently confused with several non-poisonous water snakes.

Description Dark blotches on brown or olive body. Heavy body and broad flat head.
Habitat Semiaquatic.

47 Spider or Scorpion Bites

Black Widow, Tarantula, Brown Recluse, Scorpion

Signs & Symptoms: *rigid abdominal muscles without tenderness/breathing difficulty/slurred speech/restlessness/muscle cramps/nausea, vomiting/blister at site/many other possible signs & symptoms (see next page).*

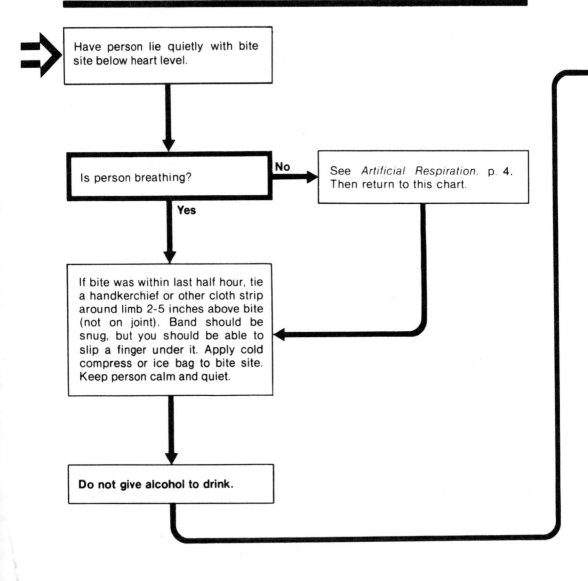

Have person lie quietly with bite site below heart level.

Is person breathing?

No → See *Artificial Respiration.* p. 4. Then return to this chart.

Yes

If bite was within last half hour, tie a handkerchief or other cloth strip around limb 2-5 inches above bite (not on joint). Band should be snug, but you should be able to slip a finger under it. Apply cold compress or ice bag to bite site. Keep person calm and quiet.

Do not give alcohol to drink.

Calm the person by talking while attending to the problem. Explain what you are doing. Try not to show anxiety; act with confidence. Your calm behavior can help to reassure the injured person.

If there are two or more rescuers, one should obtain emergency assistance while the other is following the procedures outlined below.

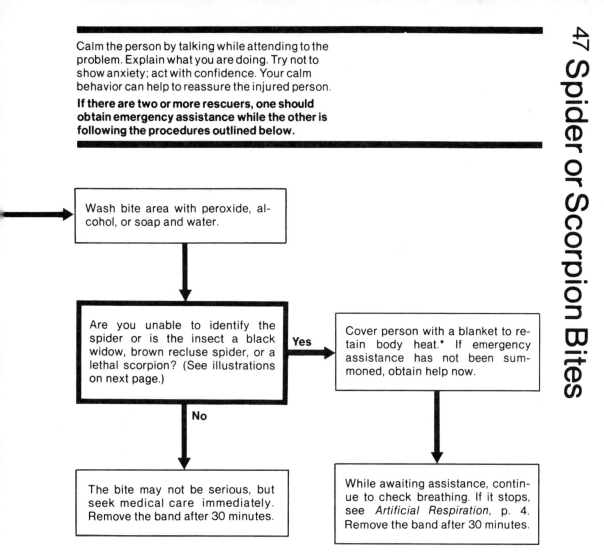

Wash bite area with peroxide, alcohol, or soap and water.

Are you unable to identify the spider or is the insect a black widow, brown recluse spider, or a lethal scorpion? (See illustrations on next page.)

Yes

Cover person with a blanket to retain body heat.* If emergency assistance has not been summoned, obtain help now.

No

The bite may not be serious, but seek medical care immediately. Remove the band after 30 minutes.

While awaiting assistance, continue to check breathing. If it stops, see *Artificial Respiration*, p. 4. Remove the band after 30 minutes.

*If weather is very warm and person's skin does not feel cool and clammy, covering will not be necessary.

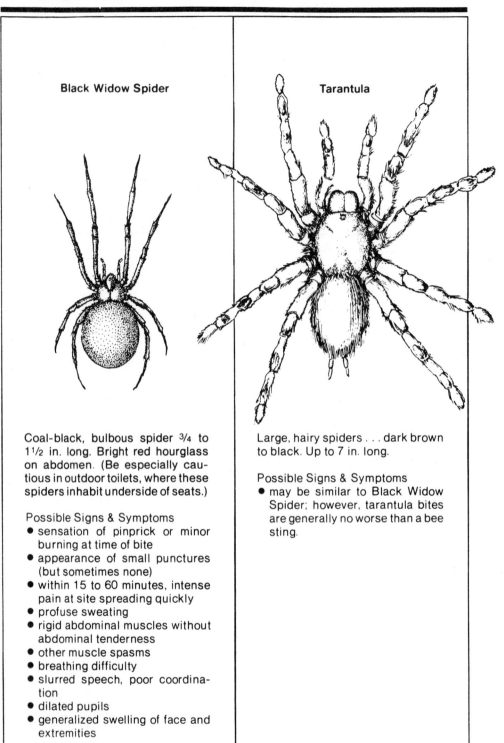

Black Widow Spider

Tarantula

Coal-black, bulbous spider ¾ to 1½ in. long. Bright red hourglass on abdomen. (Be especially cautious in outdoor toilets, where these spiders inhabit underside of seats.)

Possible Signs & Symptoms
- sensation of pinprick or minor burning at time of bite
- appearance of small punctures (but sometimes none)
- within 15 to 60 minutes, intense pain at site spreading quickly
- profuse sweating
- rigid abdominal muscles without abdominal tenderness
- other muscle spasms
- breathing difficulty
- slurred speech, poor coordination
- dilated pupils
- generalized swelling of face and extremities

Large, hairy spiders . . . dark brown to black. Up to 7 in. long.

Possible Signs & Symptoms
- may be similar to Black Widow Spider; however, tarantula bites are generally no worse than a bee sting.

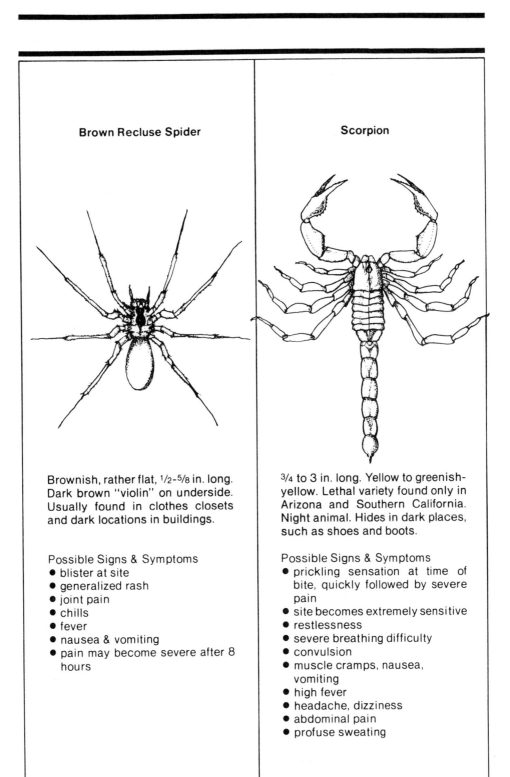

Brown Recluse Spider

Scorpion

Brownish, rather flat, 1/2-5/8 in. long. Dark brown "violin" on underside. Usually found in clothes closets and dark locations in buildings.

Possible Signs & Symptoms
- blister at site
- generalized rash
- joint pain
- chills
- fever
- nausea & vomiting
- pain may become severe after 8 hours

3/4 to 3 in. long. Yellow to greenish-yellow. Lethal variety found only in Arizona and Southern California. Night animal. Hides in dark places, such as shoes and boots.

Possible Signs & Symptoms
- prickling sensation at time of bite, quickly followed by severe pain
- site becomes extremely sensitive
- restlessness
- severe breathing difficulty
- convulsion
- muscle cramps, nausea, vomiting
- high fever
- headache, dizziness
- abdominal pain
- profuse sweating

48 Sprain or Strain

Signs & Symptoms:
Sprain (joint): swelling and discoloration of joint area/pain with movement/no deformity of the joint
Strain (muscle, ligament, or tendon): sharp, tearing pain/possible muscle spasm/possible discoloration (later)/gradual stiffening of area.

From the Signs & Symptoms listed above, identify the type of injury.

The injury is a . . .

Sprain

Remove any clothing from around the joint. Elevate the affected joint and support it with pillows, rolled blanket, or clothing.

Apply cold, wet compresses or instant cold packs for 20 minutes every 3-4 hours. Give acetaminophen (Tylenol, Datril, etc.). Follow label directions.

Keep the affected joint elevated and continue cold packs for 20 minutes every 3-4 hours.

Do swelling and pain begin to subside after several hours?

No → Continue to keep the injured part immobile and elevated. Seek medical care.

Yes

After 24 hours, wrap the joint in an elastic bandage, keeping it firm but not too tight. Person should wear this bandage for 3 or 4 days. Apply warm, wet packs to injured area for 20 minutes, 3 times a day.

Applying elastic bandage . . .

. . . using "figure-of-eight" winding

gauze pad over joint

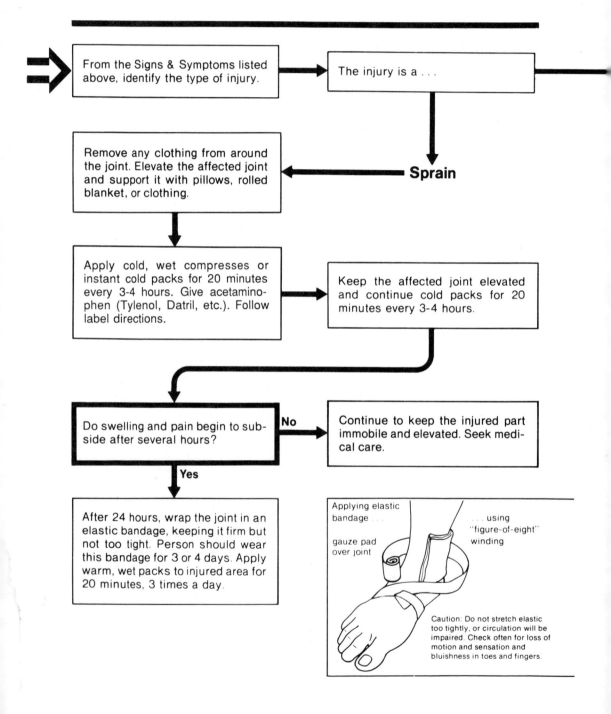

Caution: Do not stretch elastic too tightly, or circulation will be impaired. Check often for loss of motion and sensation and bluishness in toes and fingers.

Calm the person by talking while attending to the problem. Explain what you are doing. Try not to show anxiety; act with confidence. Your calm behavior can help to reassure the injured person. **If injury was the result of a vehicular or job-related accident, the person should be examined by a physician for possible additional injuries or complications.**

Strain

Is the lower back involved?

Yes → Have the person lie in a comfortable position, usually on back with knees bent.

No

Immobilize the affected part by surrounding it with rolled blankets, towels, pillows, etc.

Apply ice packs to the painful area for 15 minutes every 3-4 hours.

Apply cold, wet compresses for 20 minutes every 3-4 hours.

Give aspirin or acetaminophen (Tylenol, Datril, etc.). Follow label directions.

Continue to keep the injured part immobile. Seek medical care. ← **No** Does the pain begin to subside after several hours?

Yes

After 24 hours, apply warm, wet packs for 20 minutes every 3-4 hours. Have the person avoid any activity that produces even minor discomfort for several days.

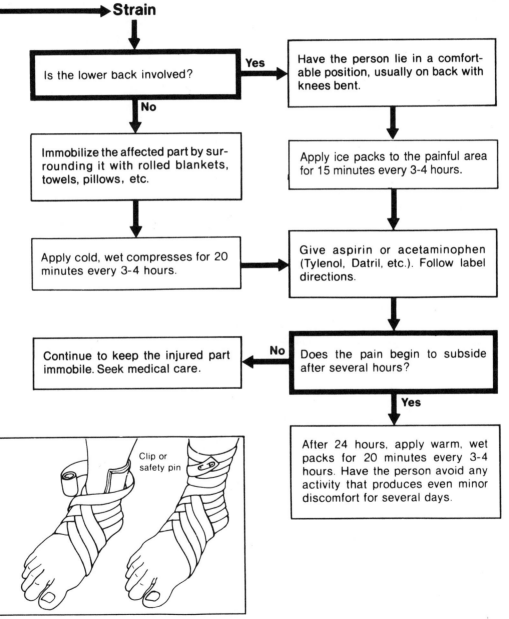

Clip or safety pin

Check for ticks on exposed areas of the body. (Don't forget to check the head and behind the ears.)

Avoid touching the tick during removal.

Do not pull tick off or apply heat since head may stay in skin.

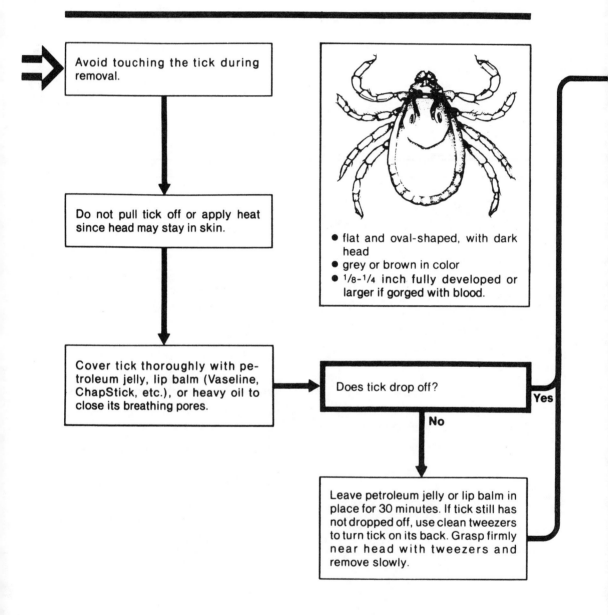

- flat and oval-shaped, with dark head
- grey or brown in color
- 1/8-1/4 inch fully developed or larger if gorged with blood.

Cover tick thoroughly with petroleum jelly, lip balm (Vaseline, ChapStick, etc.), or heavy oil to close its breathing pores.

Does tick drop off?

Yes

No

Leave petroleum jelly or lip balm in place for 30 minutes. If tick still has not dropped off, use clean tweezers to turn tick on its back. Grasp firmly near head with tweezers and remove slowly.

Calm the person by talking while attending to the problem. Explain what you are doing. Try not to show anxiety; act with confidence. Your calm behavior can help to reassure the injured person.

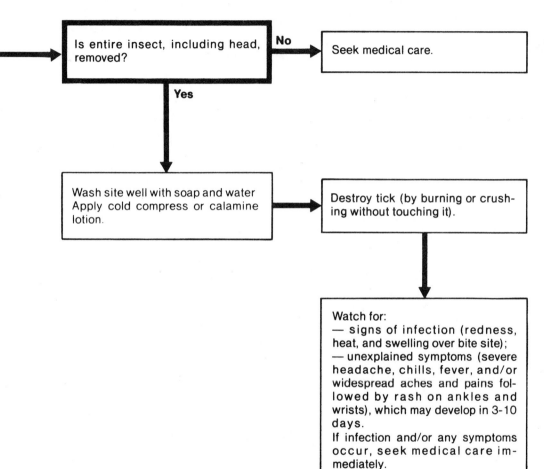

Is entire insect, including head, removed?

No → Seek medical care.

Yes

Wash site well with soap and water Apply cold compress or calamine lotion.

→ Destroy tick (by burning or crushing without touching it).

Watch for:
— signs of infection (redness, heat, and swelling over bite site);
— unexplained symptoms (severe headache, chills, fever, and/or widespread aches and pains followed by rash on ankles and wrists), which may develop in 3-10 days.
If infection and/or any symptoms occur, seek medical care immediately.

50 Deep Wound

Definition: *heavy bleeding/involvement of underlying tissues, including muscles, nerves, tendons, or major blood vessels.*

If there are two or more rescuers, one should obtain emergency assistance while the other is following the procedures outlined below.

Have the person sit or lie in a comfortable position. Immobilize the injured part, if necessary, with pillows or rolled blankets; then elevate it to help reduce bleeding. Cut clothing away from wound.

For other wounds, cover with a thick, sterile gauze pad (or other clean material) and apply gentle, firm, continuous, direct pressure with the palm of your hand.

Apply pressure with fingers and thumb to the major artery supplying blood to the wounded area (shown below).

Pressure Points

If there is a gaping facial wound, use butterfly dressing to close it (see *Minor Cuts*, p. 34). Dress with several gauze pads and four-tailed bandage or two bandages crossed and tied at top and back of head. (Be careful not to choke person.) Then see Box A on opposite page.

Do not remove the original pad; let blood soak through and begin to clot. If necessary, place additional pads over the original and continue to apply pressure for 5-10 minutes.

Does the bleeding slow down?   **No**   **Yes**

Does bleeding stop or slow down considerably?   **Yes**

No

Wrap a strip of cloth or other bandage over pad(s). Pull firmly to apply some pressure without cutting off blood circulation. Check position of fingers and thumb and reapply pressure to artery.

Calm the person by talking while attending to the problem. Explain what you are doing. Try not to show anxiety; act with confidence. Your calm behavior can help to reassure the injured person.

Bleeding Continues

Is the wound on an arm or leg?

Yes

No

Reposition the pressure bandage if necessary and repeat procedure. You have not put sufficient pressure on the appropriate pressure point.

Bleeding Slows

Leave bandage(s) in place. Add more gauze and strips. Keep affected part elevated. If bandage is very tight, it may be gradually loosened just enough to be more comfortable.

A

If a person has lost a lot of blood, feels faint, or is cold and pale, have him/her lie down. If the wound is not on the head, elevate legs from the hips on pillows or rolled blankets. If there is a head wound, elevate the head slightly. Cover the person with a blanket or clothing to retain body heat.*

If a part has been amputated, rinse it in clean water, wrap in sterile gauze or clean cloth, seal inside a plastic bag, and place on ice. Continue to control bleeding from injured limb or finger.

If emergency assistance has not been summoned, obtain help now.

While awaiting assistance, watch breathing. If it stops, see *Artificial Respiration*, p. 4. If you suspect a fracture, see p. 41.

*If weather is very warm and person's skin does not feel cool and clammy, covering will not be necessary.

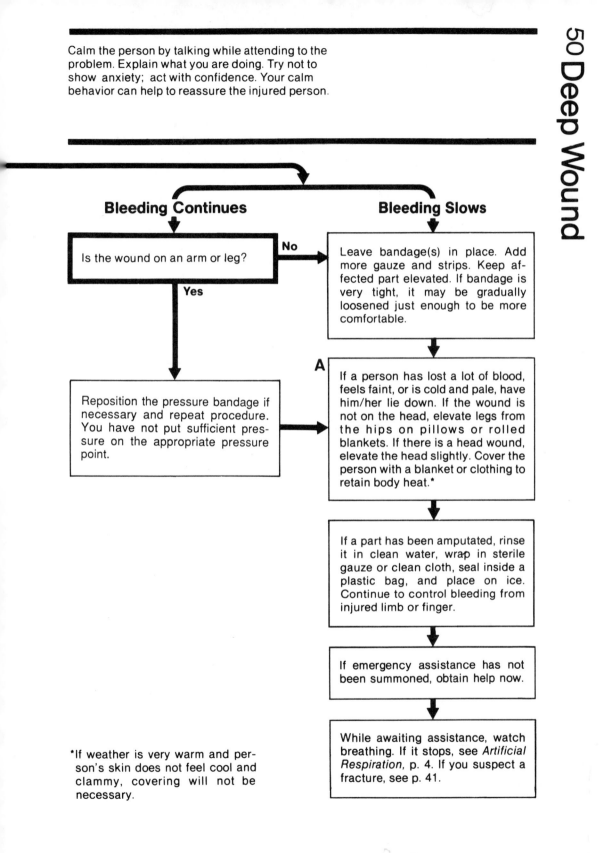

51 Cold Exposure

Signs & Symptoms: *low body temperature/ uncontrollable shivering/poor muscle coordination/shallow breathing/mental confusion/ drowsiness/numbness/possible loss of consciousness*

If there is more than one rescuer, one should obtain emergency assistance while the other is aiding the injured person.

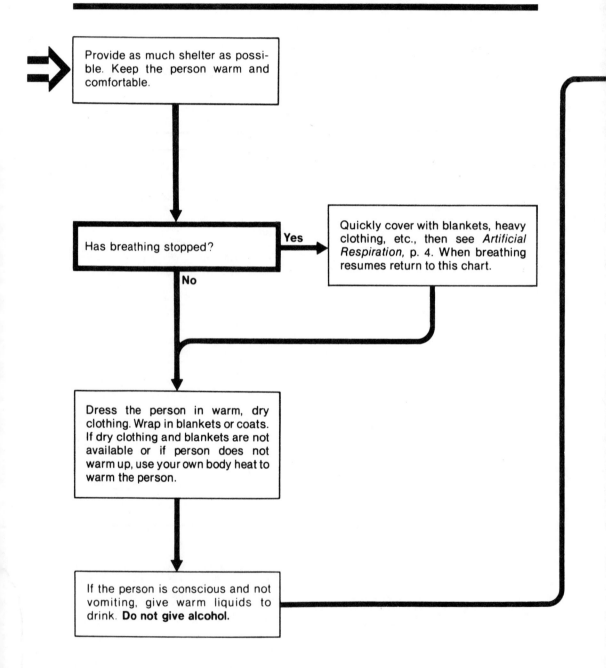

Provide as much shelter as possible. Keep the person warm and comfortable.

Has breathing stopped?

Yes

Quickly cover with blankets, heavy clothing, etc., then see *Artificial Respiration,* p. 4. When breathing resumes return to this chart.

No

Dress the person in warm, dry clothing. Wrap in blankets or coats. If dry clothing and blankets are not available or if person does not warm up, use your own body heat to warm the person.

If the person is conscious and not vomiting, give warm liquids to drink. **Do not give alcohol.**

Calm the person by talking while attending to the problem. Explain what you are doing. Try not to show anxiety; act with confidence. Your calm behavior can help to reassure the injured person.

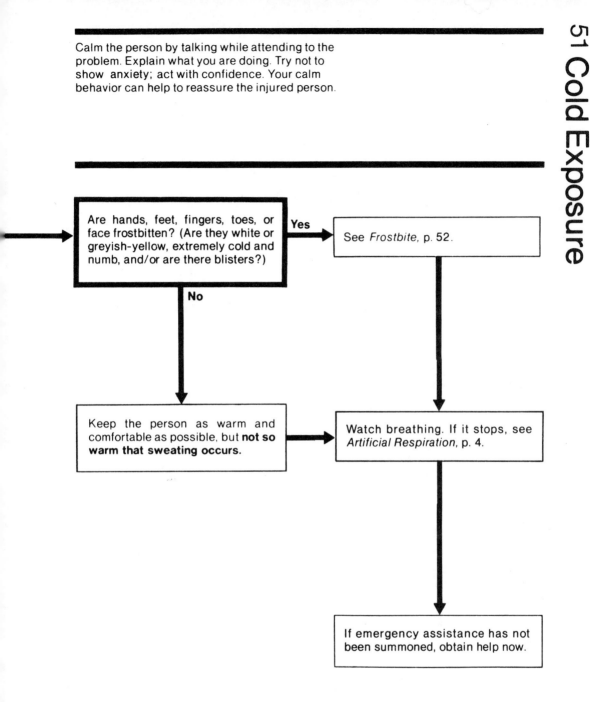

Are hands, feet, fingers, toes, or face frostbitten? (Are they white or greyish-yellow, extremely cold and numb, and/or are there blisters?)

Yes → See *Frostbite*, p. 52.

No

Keep the person as warm and comfortable as possible, but **not so warm that sweating occurs.**

Watch breathing. If it stops, see *Artificial Respiration*, p. 4.

If emergency assistance has not been summoned, obtain help now.

52 Frostbite

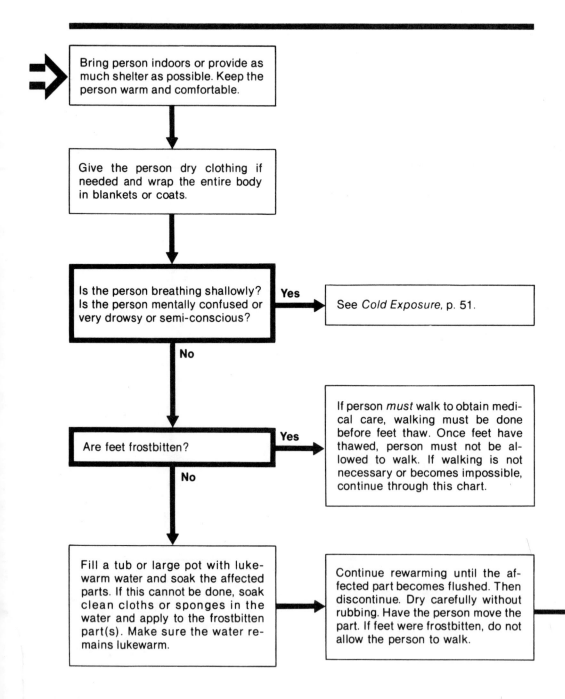

Bring person indoors or provide as much shelter as possible. Keep the person warm and comfortable.

Give the person dry clothing if needed and wrap the entire body in blankets or coats.

Is the person breathing shallowly? Is the person mentally confused or very drowsy or semi-conscious?

Yes → See *Cold Exposure*, p. 51.

No

Are feet frostbitten?

Yes → If person *must* walk to obtain medical care, walking must be done before feet thaw. Once feet have thawed, person must not be allowed to walk. If walking is not necessary or becomes impossible, continue through this chart.

No

Fill a tub or large pot with lukewarm water and soak the affected parts. If this cannot be done, soak clean cloths or sponges in the water and apply to the frostbitten part(s). Make sure the water remains lukewarm.

→ Continue rewarming until the affected part becomes flushed. Then discontinue. Dry carefully without rubbing. Have the person move the part. If feet were frostbitten, do not allow the person to walk.

Calm the person by talking while attending to the problem. Explain what you are doing. Try not to show anxiety; act with confidence. Your calm behavior can help to reassure the injured person.

Give the person dry clothes and wrap in blankets. Thaw affected part in fresh lukewarm water.

If fingers or toes were frostbitten, separate those affected with dry, sterile gauze or clean cloth. Elevate affected part(s) and protect from direct contact with bedclothes or other materials.

Keep the person as warm and comfortable as possible, but **not so warm that sweating occurs.**

Separate affected toes (or fingers) with gauze or cloth.

Give the person warm liquids to drink. **Do not give alcoholic beverages. Do not let person smoke.**

Keep the person away from sources of direct heat. If there are blisters, do not break them.

Seek medical care immediately.

53 Heat Exhaustion/ Heat Cramps

Signs & Symptoms: *cool, pale, clammy skin / fatigue and faintness/headache/ heavy sweating/ weak pulse/near-normal body temperature/ nausea. Onset is gradual.*

If person is unconscious, see *Heatstroke*, **p. 54.**

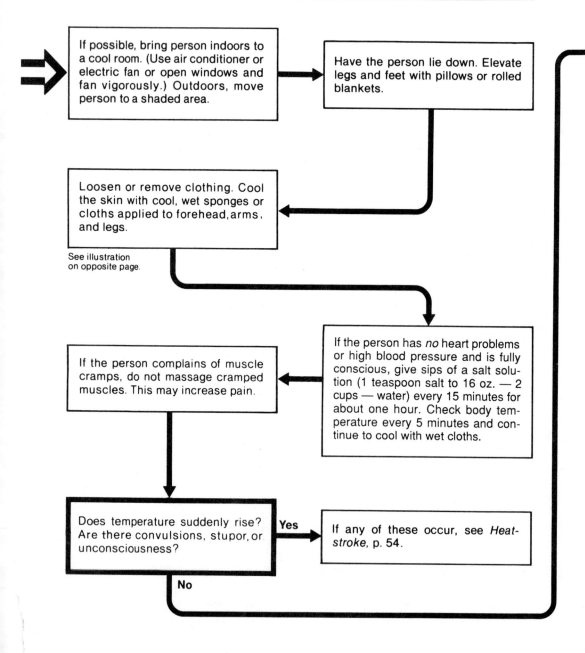

If possible, bring person indoors to a cool room. (Use air conditioner or electric fan or open windows and fan vigorously.) Outdoors, move person to a shaded area.

Have the person lie down. Elevate legs and feet with pillows or rolled blankets.

Loosen or remove clothing. Cool the skin with cool, wet sponges or cloths applied to forehead, arms, and legs.

See illustration on opposite page.

If the person has *no* heart problems or high blood pressure and is fully conscious, give sips of a salt solution (1 teaspoon salt to 16 oz. — 2 cups — water) every 15 minutes for about one hour. Check body temperature every 5 minutes and continue to cool with wet cloths.

If the person complains of muscle cramps, do not massage cramped muscles. This may increase pain.

Does temperature suddenly rise? Are there convulsions, stupor, or unconsciousness?

Yes — If any of these occur, see *Heatstroke*, p. 54.

No

Calm the person by talking while attending to the problem. Explain what you are doing. Try not to show anxiety; act with confidence. Your calm behavior can help to reassure the sick person.

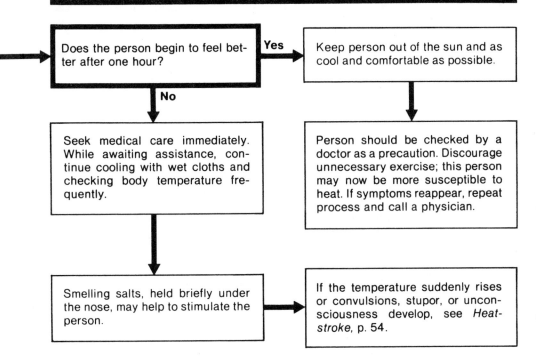

Does the person begin to feel better after one hour?

Yes → Keep person out of the sun and as cool and comfortable as possible.

No ↓

Seek medical care immediately. While awaiting assistance, continue cooling with wet cloths and checking body temperature frequently.

Person should be checked by a doctor as a precaution. Discourage unnecessary exercise; this person may now be more susceptible to heat. If symptoms reappear, repeat process and call a physician.

Smelling salts, held briefly under the nose, may help to stimulate the person.

If the temperature suddenly rises or convulsions, stupor, or unconsciousness develop, see *Heatstroke*, p. 54.

Remove all clothing. Use a sponge or cloth soaked in cool water to cool the skin. Cover lightly if at all.

Signs & Symptoms: *red, hot, dry skin/no perspira-
tion/body temperature around 106°F (or very warm
to the touch)/strong rapid pulse/stupor or unconsciousness*

**If there are two or more rescuers, one should
obtain emergency assistance while the other is
following the procedures outlined below.**

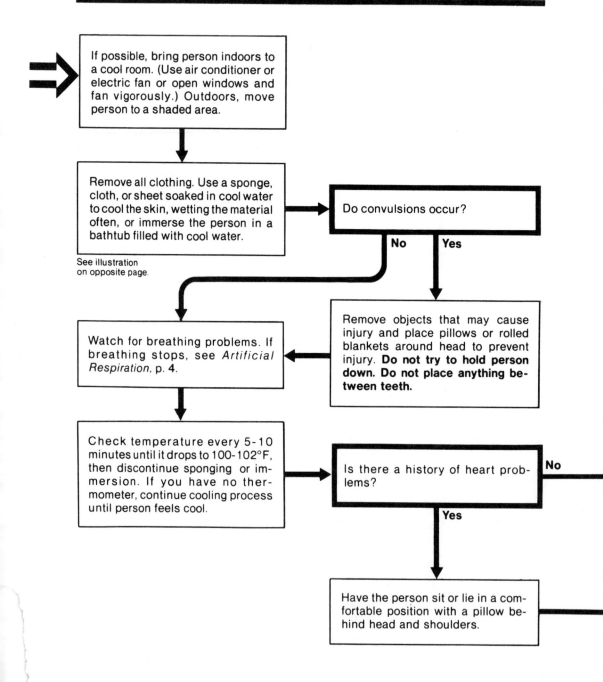

If possible, bring person indoors to a cool room. (Use air conditioner or electric fan or open windows and fan vigorously.) Outdoors, move person to a shaded area.

Remove all clothing. Use a sponge, cloth, or sheet soaked in cool water to cool the skin, wetting the material often, or immerse the person in a bathtub filled with cool water.

See illustration on opposite page.

Do convulsions occur?

No   **Yes**

Remove objects that may cause injury and place pillows or rolled blankets around head to prevent injury. **Do not try to hold person down. Do not place anything between teeth.**

Watch for breathing problems. If breathing stops, see *Artificial Respiration*, p. 4.

Check temperature every 5-10 minutes until it drops to 100-102°F, then discontinue sponging or immersion. If you have no thermometer, continue cooling process until person feels cool.

Is there a history of heart problems?   **No**

Yes

Have the person sit or lie in a comfortable position with a pillow behind head and shoulders.

Calm the person by talking while attending to the problem. Explain what you are doing. Try not to show anxiety; act with confidence. Your calm behavior can help to reassure the sick person.

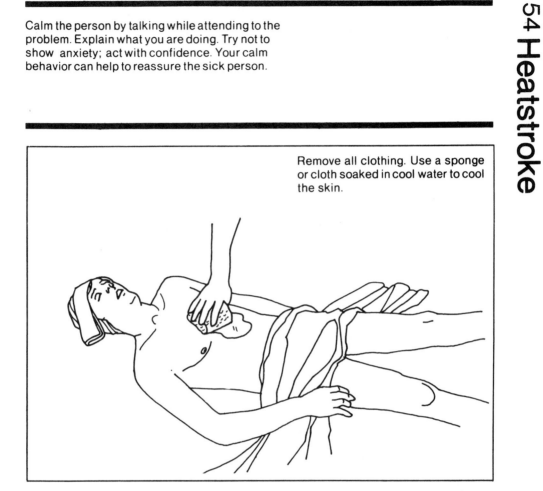

Remove all clothing. Use a sponge or cloth soaked in cool water to cool the skin.

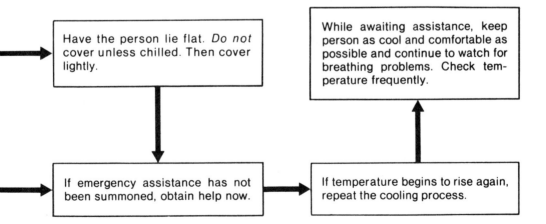

Have the person lie flat. *Do not cover unless chilled. Then cover lightly.*

While awaiting assistance, keep person as cool and comfortable as possible and continue to watch for breathing problems. Check temperature frequently.

If emergency assistance has not been summoned, obtain help now.

If temperature begins to rise again, repeat the cooling process.

55 How to Get Help Fast

Take the time *now* to fill in all the necessary information on this and the following pages so you'll be ready to give the correct information as quickly and calmly as possible in an emergency. What will the dispatcher need to know? First, the location of the accident. Besides the address, you should have available directions to your home or business from a major road. Second, your phone number in case he has to call back. Third, what happened and how many people need help. Stay on the phone until the dispatcher says it's okay to hang up.

AT HOME

1. CALL FOR HELP.

P
  H
    O
      N
        E

EMERGENCY MEDICAL SERVICES	_____
FIRE DEPARTMENT	_____
POLICE	_____
HOSPITAL	_____
POISON CONTROL CENTER	_____

2. STATE THE ADDRESS OF THE ACCIDENT OR ILLNESS AND GIVE DIRECTIONS TO IT FROM A MAJOR ROAD – INCLUDING CROSS STREETS.
    YOUR ADDRESS: _____
    DIRECTIONS TO YOUR HOUSE OR APARTMENT—SCENE OF THE ACCIDENT:
    _____
    _____
    _____
    _____

3. WHEN ASKED, GIVE YOUR PHONE NUMBER(S) AND A NEIGHBOR'S.
    YOUR PHONE NUMBER: _____
    YOUR NEIGHBOR'S: _____

4. DESCRIBE WHAT HAPPENED AND HOW MANY PEOPLE NEED HELP.

EMERGENCY TELEPHONE NUMBERS

NAMES AND NUMBERS OF NEIGHBORS TRAINED IN CPR AND FIRST AID

NAME	PHONE	TRAINING
_____	_____	_____
_____	_____	_____
_____	_____	_____
_____	_____	_____

PHYSICIANS

	NAME	OFFICE PHONE	HOME PHONE
FAMILY DOCTOR	_____	_____	_____
PEDIATRICIAN	_____	_____	_____
SPECIALIST(S)	_____	_____	_____
	_____	_____	_____
	_____	_____	_____
DENTIST	_____	_____	_____

HOSPITAL EMERGENCY ROOM _____

DRUGSTORE _____

HUSBAND'S PHONE AT WORK_____**WIFE'S PHONE AT WORK**_____

OTHER FAMILY MEMBERS' NUMBERS

NAME	WORK/SCHOOL	PHONE
_____	_____	_____
_____	_____	_____
_____	_____	_____
_____	_____	_____

NEIGHBORS AND FRIENDS

NAME	ADDRESS	PHONE
_____	_____	_____
_____	_____	_____
_____	_____	_____
_____	_____	_____

TAXI _____

AT WORK

1. CALL FOR HELP.
   - **EMERGENCY MEDICAL SERVICES** _____
   - **COMPANY MEDICAL ROOM** _____
   - **FIRE DEPARTMENT** _____
   - **POLICE** _____
   - **PERSONNEL DEPARTMENT** _____
   - **COMPANY SECURITY** _____
   - **SUPERVISOR** _____

2. STATE THE ADDRESS AND LOCATION OF THE COMPANY, INCLUDING CROSS STREETS AND SPECIFIC DIRECTIONS TO YOUR DEPARTMENT FROM THE MAIN ENTRANCE.
   - **YOUR COMPANY'S ADDRESS:** _____
   - **DIRECTIONS TO YOUR COMPANY:** _____
   - _____
   - _____
   - _____

DIRECTIONS TO YOUR DEPARTMENT: _____

_____

_____

_____

3. GIVE YOUR PHONE NUMBER AND THE NUMBER OF A NEARBY PHONE.
   YOUR PHONE NUMBER AND EXTENSION: _____
   PHONE NUMBER AND EXTENSION OF NEARBY PHONE (list location): _____

_____

4. DESCRIBE WHAT HAPPENED AND HOW MANY PEOPLE NEED HELP.

EMPLOYEES TRAINED IN FIRST AID AND/OR CPR

NAME	DEPARTMENT	PHONE	TRAINING
_____	_____	_____	_____
_____	_____	_____	_____
_____	_____	_____	_____
_____	_____	_____	_____

ON THE ROAD

1. CALL FOR HELP.

	EMERGENCY MEDICAL SERVICES	FIRE	POLICE
HOMETOWN	_____	___	___
AREAS YOU VISIT	_____	___	___
REGULARLY	_____	___	___
	_____	___	___
	_____	___	___

EMERGENCY PHONE NUMBERS

AUTO CLUB_____

TOWING SERVICES _____

AUTO REPAIR_____

TAXI _____

AUTOMOBILE INSURANCE COMPANY _____

   POLICY NUMBER _____

2. STATE THE LOCATION OF THE ACCIDENT, GIVING DIRECTIONS FROM MAJOR ROAD, INCLUDING CROSS STREETS.

3. GIVE YOUR NUMBER.

4. DESCRIBE WHAT HAPPENED AND HOW MANY PEOPLE NEED HELP. STAY ON THE LINE UNTIL DISPATCHER SAYS IT'S ALL RIGHT TO HANG UP!!!